THE BLOOD TYPE O DIET COOKBOOK

A Comprehensive Culinary Companion Tailored to Enhance Health, Energy, and Well-Being through the Blood Type O Diet

Linda M. Craig

Copyright © [2024] [Linda M. Craig]

Table of content

Chapter One: Understanding the Blood Type O Diet

Introduction to the Blood Type O Diet

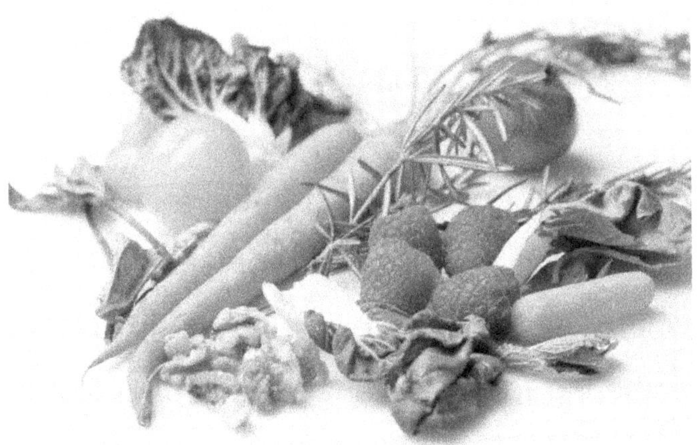

The Blood Type O Diet is based on the principle that different blood types evolved at different times in human history, and therefore, each blood type is better suited to certain types of foods.

Understanding Blood Type O:

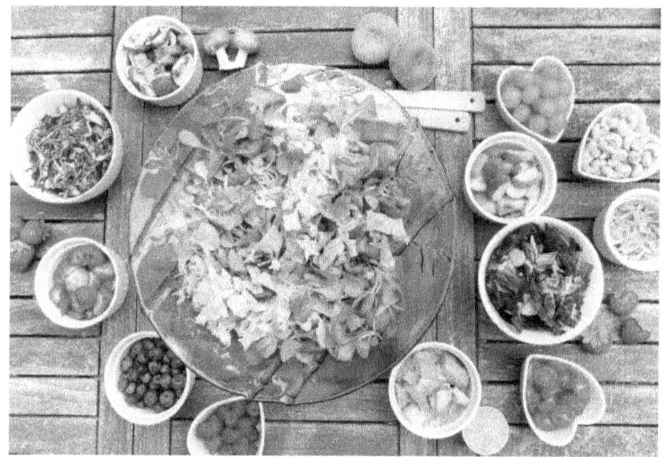

Blood type O is believed to have originated in ancient hunter-gatherer populations, where individuals relied on hunting and gathering for sustenance. According to the Blood Type O Diet theory, people with type O blood have a robust digestive system and produce higher levels of stomach acid and digestive enzymes, making them better suited to digest and metabolize animal proteins.

Principles of the Blood Type O Diet:

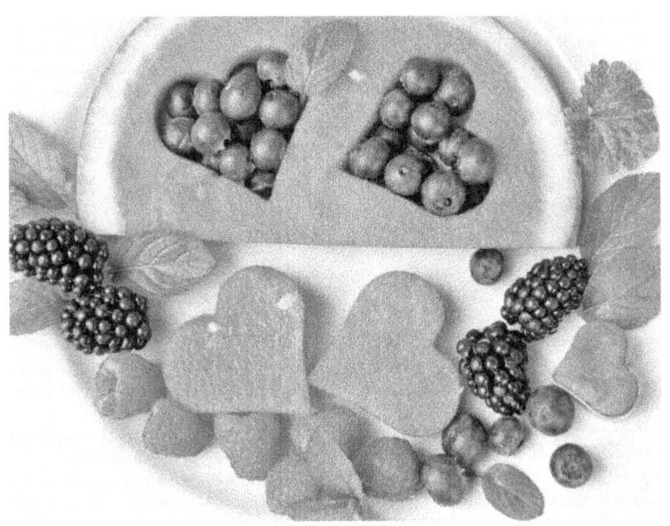

The primary principles of the Blood Type O Diet revolve around consuming a diet rich in lean proteins, such as meat, fish, and poultry, and limiting grains and dairy products. The diet also emphasizes the importance of incorporating high-intensity aerobic exercise into one's lifestyle to support overall health and weight management.

Benefits of the Blood Type O Diet:

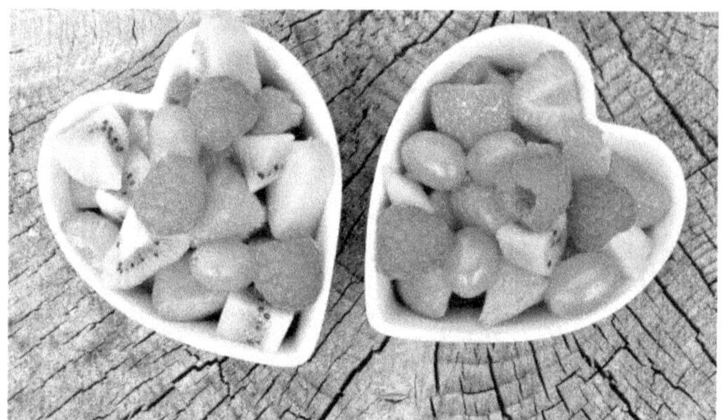

Proponents of the Blood Type O Diet claim that adhering to this eating plan can lead to numerous health benefits, including improved digestion, increased energy levels, weight loss, and reduced risk of chronic diseases such as heart disease and diabetes. By aligning dietary choices with one's blood type, individuals are purported to experience enhanced overall well-being and vitality.

Scientific Evidence and Criticisms:

While some anecdotal evidence supports the efficacy of the Blood Type O Diet, scientific research validating its principles is limited. Critics argue that the diet lacks scientific basis and that individual variations in genetics, lifestyle, and overall health may have a more significant impact on dietary requirements than blood type alone. Additionally, the restrictive nature of the diet, particularly in its avoidance of certain food groups, may pose challenges in meeting essential nutrient needs for some individuals.

Getting Started with the Blood Type O Diet:

Before embarking on the Blood Type O Diet, it is essential for individuals to consult with a healthcare professional or registered dietitian to ensure that it is appropriate for their individual health needs and goals. Additionally, transitioning to this eating plan may require careful meal planning and food substitutions to accommodate dietary restrictions and preferences while still meeting nutritional requirements.

The Introduction to the Blood Type O Diet provides readers with an overview of the principles and rationale behind this unique dietary approach. While further research is needed to fully elucidate its efficacy and suitability for individuals of blood type O, many proponents find success in aligning their dietary choices with their evolutionary heritage. By understanding the principles and potential benefits of the Blood Type O Diet, individuals can make informed decisions about their dietary habits and overall health and well-being.

Benefits of Eating According to Your Blood Type

Eating according to your blood type is a concept popularized by the Blood Type Diet, which suggests that individuals can optimize their health and well-being by tailoring their diet to their specific blood type. While this approach has garnered both praise and skepticism, proponents argue that adhering to a diet aligned with one's blood type can offer a range of benefits. Below are the key benefits associated with eating according to your blood type:

1. Enhanced Digestion and Nutrient Absorption:

The Blood Type Diet posits that certain foods may be better tolerated and more easily digested by individuals based on their blood type. By eliminating foods that are incompatible with one's blood type, proponents claim that individuals can reduce digestive discomfort, such as bloating, gas, and indigestion, and improve nutrient absorption, leading to better overall health.

2. Increased Energy Levels:

Advocates of the Blood Type Diet suggest that eating foods compatible with one's blood type can lead to increased energy levels and overall vitality. By consuming a diet rich in foods that are easily metabolized and utilized by the body, individuals may experience sustained energy throughout the day, improved focus, and enhanced physical performance.

3. Weight Management and Body Composition:

Another purported benefit of eating according to your blood type is improved weight management and body composition. The diet emphasizes the consumption of whole, nutrient-dense foods while limiting or avoiding processed foods, refined sugars, and artificial additives. By promoting a balanced intake of protein, carbohydrates, and fats tailored to individual blood types, proponents claim that the diet can support healthy weight loss, maintenance, and muscle mass development.

4. Reduced Risk of Chronic Diseases:

Some proponents suggest that aligning dietary choices with one's blood type may reduce the risk of developing chronic diseases, such as heart disease, diabetes, and certain autoimmune conditions. By eliminating foods that may trigger inflammation or immune responses in susceptible individuals, the Blood Type Diet aims to support overall health and mitigate disease risk factors.

5. Personalized Approach to Nutrition:

One of the primary benefits of the Blood Type Diet is its personalized approach to nutrition. By considering individual genetic factors, proponents argue that the diet can provide tailored dietary recommendations that optimize health outcomes and promote overall well-being. This personalized approach may empower individuals to make informed dietary choices that resonate with their unique physiology and health goals.

Conclusion:

While the benefits of eating according to your blood type are often touted by proponents of the Blood Type Diet, it is essential to approach this dietary approach with a critical eye and consult with a healthcare professional or registered dietitian before making significant changes to your eating habits. While some individuals may experience positive outcomes from following the Blood Type Diet, others may find it restrictive or lacking in scientific evidence. Ultimately, the decision to adopt this dietary approach should be based on individual preferences, health goals, and nutritional needs.

Successfully following the Blood Type O Diet requires dedication, planning, and understanding of its principles. Here are some tips to help individuals achieve success on this dietary plan:

1. Educate Yourself About Your Blood Type:

Begin by learning about the characteristics and nutritional recommendations specific to blood type O. Understanding why certain foods are recommended or restricted can help you make informed choices and stay motivated to adhere to the diet.

2. Stock Up on Blood Type O-Friendly Foods:

Fill your pantry and refrigerator with foods that align with the Blood Type O Diet guidelines. Focus on lean proteins such as beef, lamb, poultry, and fish, as well as fruits, vegetables, and healthy fats like olive oil and nuts.

3. Plan Your Meals and Snacks:

Take time to plan your meals and snacks in advance to ensure they comply with the Blood Type O Diet. Consider batch cooking and meal prepping to have convenient, blood type O-friendly options readily available throughout the week.

4. Experiment with Recipes and Cooking Methods:

Explore different recipes and cooking methods to keep your meals interesting and flavorful. Experiment with herbs, spices, and marinades to enhance the taste of lean proteins and vegetables while avoiding ingredients that are not compatible with blood type O.

5. Listen to Your Body:

Pay attention to how your body responds to different foods and adjust your diet accordingly. While the Blood Type O Diet provides general guidelines, individual tolerances and preferences may vary. If certain foods cause discomfort or adverse reactions, consider eliminating or minimizing them from your diet.

6. Stay Hydrated:

Drink plenty of water throughout the day to support digestion, hydration, and overall health. Herbal teas and sparkling water can also be enjoyed as refreshing alternatives to sugary beverages and caffeinated drinks.

7. Incorporate Regular Exercise:

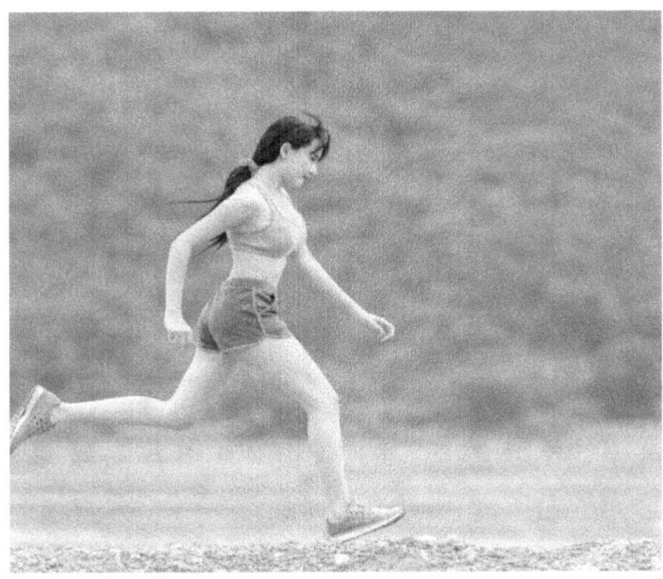

Engage in regular physical activity, focusing on high-intensity aerobic exercises such as running, cycling, or swimming. Exercise not only supports weight management but also promotes cardiovascular health and overall well-being, complementing the benefits of the Blood Type O Diet.

8. Practice Mindful Eating:

Be mindful of your eating habits and strive to eat slowly, savoring each bite and paying attention to hunger and fullness cues. Mindful eating can help prevent overeating, promote better digestion, and enhance your overall dining experience.

9. Seek Support and Accountability:

Connect with others following the Blood Type O Diet for support, encouragement, and recipe ideas. Consider joining online forums, social media groups, or local meetups to share experiences and stay motivated on your dietary journey.

10. Be Patient and Flexible:

Lastly, be patient with yourself and recognize that adopting a new dietary approach takes time and adjustment. Embrace the process of discovering what works best for your body, and be open to making modifications to your diet as needed to achieve long-term success on the Blood Type O Diet.

By incorporating these tips into your lifestyle, you can maximize your chances of success and experience the potential benefits of the Blood Type O Diet in supporting your overall health and well-being.

Chapter Two: Breakfast Recipes

Energizing Smoothie Bowls

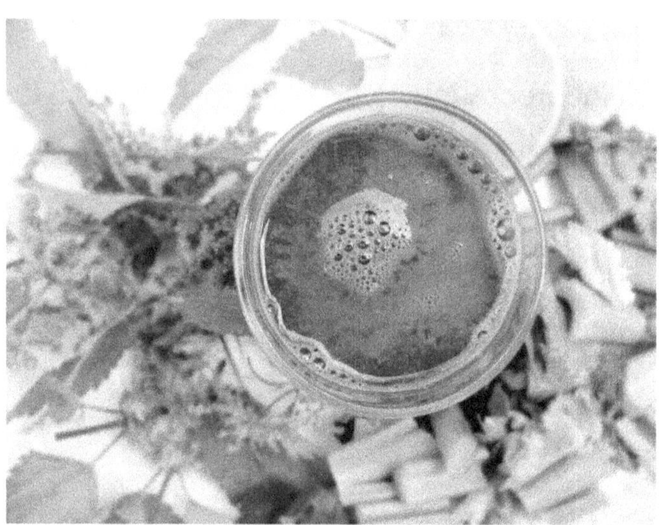

Smoothie bowls have become a popular breakfast and snack option for individuals looking for a nutritious and convenient meal that can be customized to suit their tastes and dietary preferences. In this chapter, we explore how to create energizing smoothie bowls specifically tailored to individuals following the Blood Type O Diet.

1. Understanding Blood Type O-Friendly Ingredients:

When preparing smoothie bowls for blood type O individuals, it's important to focus on ingredients that align with the diet's principles. This includes incorporating protein-rich ingredients such as whey protein powder, Greek yogurt, or almond butter to support satiety and muscle repair.

2. Selecting Blood Type O-Friendly Fruits and Vegetables:

Choose fruits and vegetables that are compatible with the Blood Type O Diet, such as berries (especially blueberries and strawberries), bananas, pineapple, spinach, and kale. These ingredients provide essential vitamins, minerals, and antioxidants while satisfying sweet cravings.

3. Incorporating Healthy Fats and Fiber:

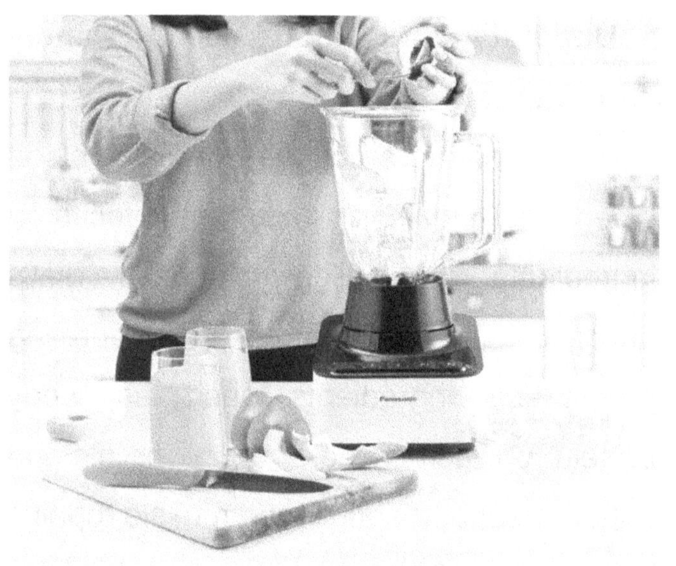

To enhance the nutritional profile and satiety of smoothie bowls, include sources of healthy fats and fiber such as avocado, chia seeds, flaxseeds, or unsweetened coconut flakes. These ingredients provide sustained energy and promote digestive health.

4. Adding Liquid Base:

For the liquid base of your smoothie bowls, opt for blood type O-friendly options such as almond milk, coconut water, or water. Avoid dairy milk and fruit juices, which may not be well-tolerated by some individuals following the Blood Type O Diet.

5. Boosting Flavor and Nutrition:

Incorporate flavor-enhancing ingredients such as cinnamon, vanilla extract, ginger, or fresh mint to elevate the taste of your smoothie bowls without adding unnecessary sugar or calories. Additionally, consider adding superfood powders like spirulina or wheatgrass for an extra nutritional boost.

6. Toppings and Garnishes:

Experiment with a variety of toppings and garnishes to add texture, flavor, and visual appeal to your smoothie bowls. Blood type O-friendly options include sliced almonds, pumpkin seeds, hemp hearts, cacao nibs, and unsweetened shredded coconut.

7. Balancing Macronutrients:

To create a well-rounded and satisfying smoothie bowl, aim to balance macronutrients by including a combination of protein, carbohydrates, and fats. This helps stabilize blood sugar levels, prevent energy crashes, and promote sustained energy throughout the day.

8. Portion Control and Moderation:

While smoothie bowls can be a nutritious addition to your diet, it's important to practice portion control and moderation, especially if you're watching your calorie intake or trying to manage your weight. Pay attention to portion sizes and avoid loading your smoothie bowl with excessive toppings or sweeteners.

9. Customizing to Suit Individual Preferences:

One of the benefits of smoothie bowls is their versatility, allowing individuals to customize ingredients and flavors to suit their tastes and dietary needs. Experiment with different combinations of fruits, vegetables, proteins, and toppings to create your perfect blood type O-friendly smoothie bowl.

10. Enjoying Mindfully:

Lastly, savor your smoothie bowl mindfully, taking time to appreciate the flavors, textures, and nourishment it provides. Sit down, chew slowly, and pay attention to your hunger and fullness cues to promote digestion and enjoyment of your meal.

By following these guidelines and experimenting with different ingredients and flavor combinations, you can create delicious and energizing smoothie bowls that align with the principles of the Blood Type O Diet, supporting your health and well-being.

Protein-Packed Omelettes

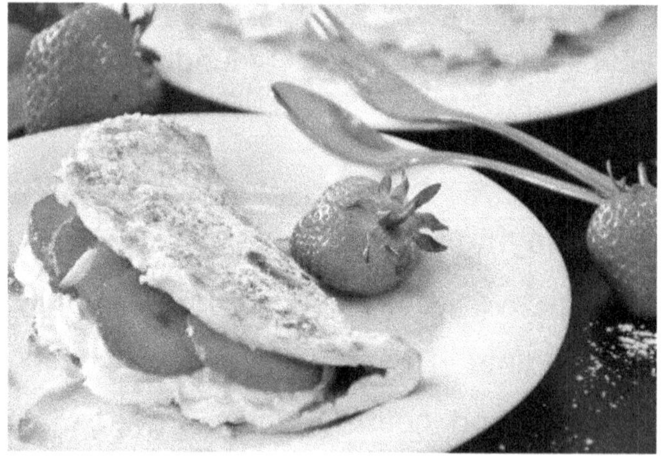

Omelettes are a versatile and nutritious dish that can be customized to suit the preferences and dietary needs of individuals following the Blood Type O Diet. In this chapter, we explore how to create protein-packed omelettes that provide essential nutrients while aligning with the principles of the diet.

1. Choosing High-Protein Ingredients:

Start by selecting protein-rich ingredients that are compatible with the Blood Type O Diet. Good options include eggs, lean meats such as chicken, turkey, or beef, as well as seafood like salmon or shrimp. These ingredients provide the necessary protein to support muscle repair and satiety.

2. Incorporating Blood Type O-Friendly Vegetables:

Add a variety of vegetables to your omelette to increase fiber, vitamins, and minerals. Suitable options for blood type O individuals include spinach, kale, bell peppers, onions, mushrooms, and tomatoes. These vegetables not only enhance the flavor and texture of the omelette but also contribute to overall health and well-being.

3. Including Healthy Fats:

Incorporate sources of healthy fats into your omelette to promote satiety and support brain health. Avocado, olive oil, and coconut oil are excellent choices for blood type O individuals. Avoid using butter or margarine, which may not be well-tolerated by some individuals on the Blood Type O Diet.

4. Avoiding Dairy:

For individuals following the Blood Type O Diet, it's advisable to limit or avoid dairy products, including cheese and milk. Instead, focus on incorporating non-dairy sources of calcium and protein, such as leafy greens, tofu, or fortified plant-based milk alternatives.

5. Experimenting with Herbs and Spices: Enhance the flavor of your omelette with herbs, spices, and seasonings that are compatible with the Blood Type O Diet. Consider using fresh herbs like parsley, basil, or cilantro, as well as spices such as garlic, turmeric, or cayenne pepper to add depth and complexity to your dish.

6. Balancing Macronutrients:

Ensure that your omelette provides a balance of macronutrients, including protein, carbohydrates, and fats, to support overall health and energy levels. Aim to include a variety of ingredients to create a well-rounded and satisfying meal.

7. Cooking Methods:

When preparing protein-packed omelettes, opt for healthier cooking methods such as sautéing or baking instead of frying. Use minimal oil or cooking spray to reduce unnecessary added fats and calories.

8. Customizing to Suit Individual Preferences:

Omelettes are highly customizable, allowing individuals to tailor ingredients and flavors to their liking. Experiment with different combinations of proteins, vegetables, and seasonings to create your perfect blood type O-friendly omelette.

9. Pairing with Blood Type O-Friendly Sides:

Serve your protein-packed omelette with blood type O-friendly sides such as sliced avocado, mixed greens, or sweet potato hash. These options complement the omelette and provide additional nutrients and fiber.

10. Enjoying Mindfully:

Sit down and enjoy your protein-packed omelette mindfully, taking time to savor each bite and appreciate the nourishment it provides. Eat slowly, chew thoroughly, and listen to your body's hunger and fullness cues to promote digestion and satisfaction.

By following these guidelines and incorporating protein-packed omelettes into your diet, you can enjoy a delicious and nutritious meal that supports your health and well-being on the Blood Type O Diet.

Hearty Breakfast Hash

A hearty breakfast hash is a satisfying and nutritious dish that can be enjoyed by individuals following the Blood Type O Diet. In this chapter, we explore how to create a flavorful and protein-rich breakfast hash that aligns with the principles of the diet.

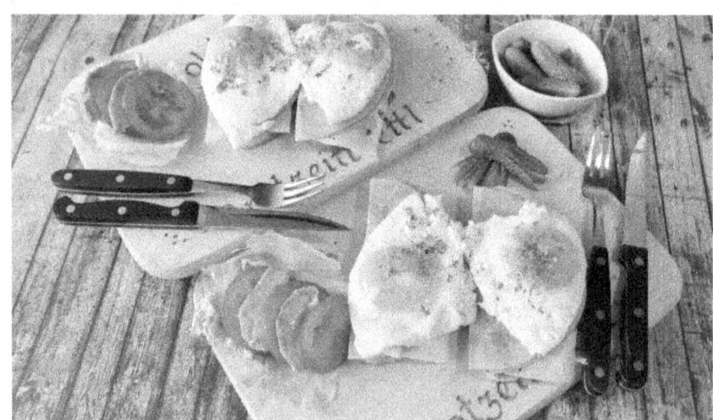

1. Selecting Blood Type O-Friendly Proteins:

Start by choosing protein sources that are compatible with the Blood Type O Diet. Opt for lean meats such as turkey, chicken, or beef, as well as seafood like salmon or shrimp. These protein-rich ingredients provide essential nutrients while supporting muscle repair and satiety.

2. Incorporating Blood Type O-Friendly Vegetables:

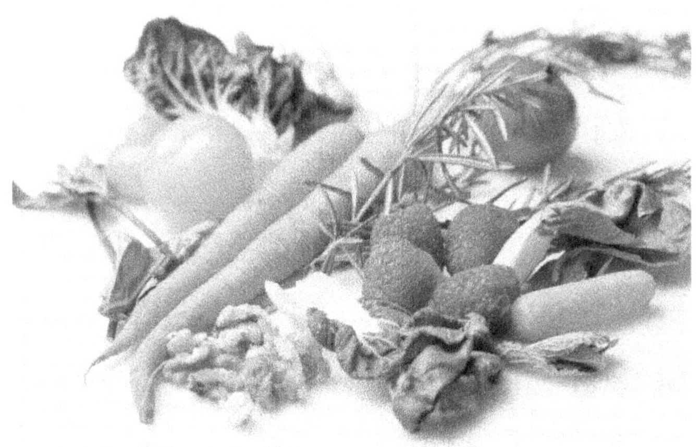

Add a variety of vegetables to your breakfast hash to increase fiber, vitamins, and minerals. Suitable options for blood type O individuals include sweet potatoes, onions, bell peppers, spinach, kale, and mushrooms. These vegetables add flavor, texture, and nutritional value to the dish.

3. Using Healthy Cooking Fats:
Choose healthy fats such as olive oil, avocado oil, or coconut oil for cooking your breakfast hash. These fats provide essential fatty acids and help enhance the flavor and texture of the dish. Avoid using butter or margarine, which may not be well-tolerated by some individuals on the Blood Type O Diet.

4. Balancing Flavors and Seasonings:
Season your breakfast hash with herbs, spices, and seasonings that are compatible

with the Blood Type O Diet. Consider using garlic, onion powder, paprika, cumin, or rosemary to add depth and complexity to the dish. Experiment with different flavor combinations to suit your taste preferences.

5. Cooking Methods:

When preparing a hearty breakfast hash, aim to sauté or roast the ingredients to develop rich flavors and textures. Use a non-stick skillet or baking sheet to minimize the need for excessive cooking fats and prevent sticking.

6. Adding Blood Type O-Friendly Extras:

Enhance the nutritional profile of your breakfast hash by incorporating blood type O-friendly extras such as diced avocado, chopped nuts or seeds, or a drizzle of hot sauce. These additions provide additional nutrients, flavor, and texture to the dish.

7. Customizing to Suit Individual Preferences:

Breakfast hash is a versatile dish that can be customized to suit individual preferences and dietary needs. Experiment with different combinations of proteins, vegetables, and seasonings to create your perfect blood type O-friendly breakfast hash.

8. Pairing with Blood Type O-Friendly Sides:

Serve your hearty breakfast hash with blood type O-friendly sides such as sliced fruit, mixed greens, or a side of steamed vegetables. These options complement the flavors of the hash and provide additional nutrients and fiber.

9. Enjoying Mindfully:

Sit down and enjoy your hearty breakfast hash mindfully, taking time to savor each bite and appreciate the nourishment it provides. Eat slowly, chew thoroughly, and listen to your body's hunger and fullness cues to promote digestion and satisfaction.

10. Meal Prep and Storage Tips:
Consider preparing a batch of breakfast hash ahead of time and storing individual portions in the refrigerator or freezer for quick and convenient meals throughout the week. Reheat leftovers in a skillet or microwave until heated through.

By following these guidelines and incorporating hearty breakfast hash into your diet, you can enjoy a delicious and nutritious meal that supports your health and well-being on the Blood Type O Diet.

Chapter Three: Lunchtime Favorites

Grilled Chicken Salad with Balsamic Vinaigrette

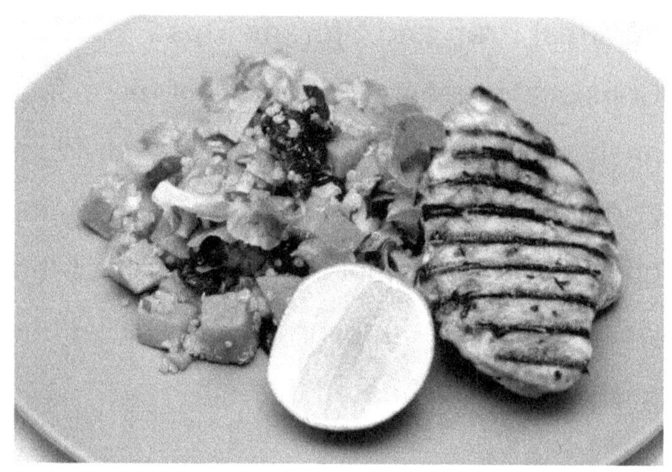

Grilled chicken salad with balsamic vinaigrette is a delicious and nutritious dish that is well-suited for individuals following the Blood Type O Diet. In this chapter, we explore how to prepare a flavorful salad using blood type O-friendly ingredients and a homemade balsamic vinaigrette dressing.

1. Selecting Blood Type O-Friendly Ingredients:

Choose ingredients for your grilled chicken salad that align with the Blood Type O Diet. Focus on incorporating lean proteins such as grilled chicken breast, which provides essential nutrients while supporting muscle repair and satiety.

2. Incorporating Blood Type O-Friendly Vegetables:

Add a variety of vegetables to your salad to increase fiber, vitamins, and minerals. Suitable options for blood type O individuals include mixed greens, spinach, tomatoes, cucumbers, bell peppers, red onions, and avocado. These vegetables add color, texture, and nutritional value to the salad.

3. Grilling Chicken:

Marinate chicken breasts in a blood type O-friendly marinade, such as olive oil, lemon juice, garlic, and herbs. Grill the chicken until cooked through, then slice or dice it and allow it to cool slightly before adding it to the salad.

4. Preparing Balsamic Vinaigrette Dressing:

Make a homemade balsamic vinaigrette dressing using blood type O-friendly ingredients such as extra virgin olive oil, balsamic vinegar, Dijon mustard, garlic, and herbs. Whisk the ingredients together in a bowl until well combined, then drizzle the dressing over the salad just before serving.

5. Adding Texture and Flavor:

Enhance the flavor and texture of your grilled chicken salad by incorporating additional blood type O-friendly ingredients such as toasted nuts or seeds, crumbled feta cheese (if tolerated), or dried cranberries. These additions add crunch, creaminess, and sweetness to the salad.

6. Balancing Macronutrients:

Ensure that your grilled chicken salad provides a balance of macronutrients, including protein, carbohydrates, and fats, to support overall health and energy levels. Aim to include a variety of ingredients to create a well-rounded and satisfying meal.

7. Customizing to Suit Individual Preferences:

Grilled chicken salad is highly customizable, allowing individuals to tailor ingredients and flavors to their liking. Experiment with different combinations of vegetables, proteins, and toppings to create your perfect blood type O-friendly salad.

8. Pairing with Blood Type O-Friendly Sides:

Serve your grilled chicken salad with blood type O-friendly sides such as whole grain bread, quinoa, or brown rice. These options complement the flavors of the salad and provide additional nutrients and fiber.

9. Enjoying Mindfully:

Sit down and enjoy your grilled chicken salad mindfully, taking time to savor each bite and appreciate the nourishment it provides. Chew slowly, and listen to your body's hunger and fullness cues to promote digestion and satisfaction.

10. Meal Prep and Storage Tips:

Consider preparing a batch of grilled chicken salad ahead of time and storing individual portions in airtight containers in the refrigerator for quick and convenient meals throughout the week. Keep the dressing separate until ready to serve to prevent the salad from becoming soggy.

By following these guidelines and incorporating grilled chicken salad with balsamic vinaigrette into your diet, you can enjoy a delicious and nutritious meal that supports your health and well-being on the Blood Type O Diet.

Turkey and Avocado Wrap

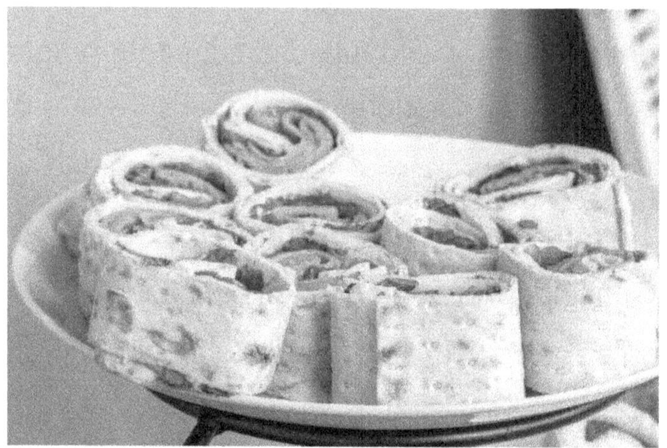

Turkey and avocado wrap is a nutritious and satisfying meal option that aligns with the principles of the Blood Type O Diet. In this chapter, we explore how to create a flavorful and protein-rich wrap using blood type O-friendly ingredients.

1. Choosing Blood Type O-Friendly Protein:

Select turkey breast as the primary protein for your wrap. Turkey is a lean source of protein that provides essential nutrients while supporting muscle repair and satiety. Opt for organic or free-range turkey whenever possible for the highest quality.

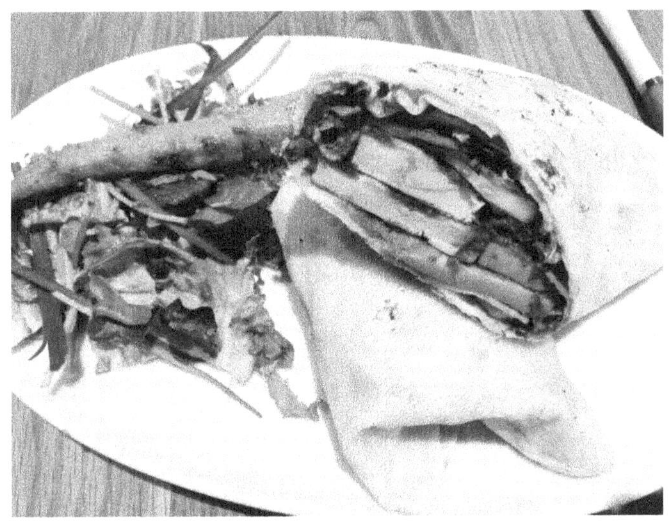

2. Incorporating Blood Type O-Friendly Vegetables:

Add a variety of vegetables to your wrap to increase fiber, vitamins, and minerals. Suitable options for blood type O individuals include leafy greens, tomatoes, cucumbers, bell peppers, and red onions. These vegetables add color, texture, and nutritional value to the wrap.

3. Including Healthy Fats:

Incorporate avocado slices into your wrap to add healthy fats, creaminess, and flavor. Avocado is rich in monounsaturated fats, which are beneficial for heart health and satiety. It also provides essential nutrients such as potassium, vitamin K, and folate.

4. Choosing Blood Type O-Friendly Wraps:

Select whole grain or sprouted grain wraps for your turkey and avocado wrap. These options are higher in fiber and nutrients compared to traditional white wraps, providing sustained energy and supporting digestive health.

5. Adding Flavorful Condiments:

Enhance the flavor of your wrap with blood type O-friendly condiments such as Dijon mustard, hummus, or pesto. These additions add depth and complexity to the wrap without adding unnecessary calories or artificial ingredients.

6. Balancing Macronutrients:

Ensure that your turkey and avocado wrap provides a balance of macronutrients, including protein, carbohydrates, and fats, to support overall health and energy levels. Aim to include a variety of ingredients to create a well-rounded and satisfying meal.

7. Customizing to Suit Individual Preferences:

Turkey and avocado wraps are highly customizable, allowing individuals to tailor ingredients and flavors to their liking. Experiment with different combinations of proteins, vegetables, and condiments to create your perfect blood type O-friendly wrap.

8. Pairing with Blood Type O-Friendly Sides:

Serve your turkey and avocado wrap with blood type O-friendly sides such as mixed greens, sliced fruit, or a side of steamed vegetables. These options complement the flavors of the wrap and provide additional nutrients and fiber.

9. Enjoying Mindfully:

Sit down and enjoy your turkey and avocado wrap mindfully, taking time to savor each bite and appreciate the nourishment it provides. Chew slowly, and listen to your body's hunger and fullness cues to promote digestion and satisfaction.

10. Meal Prep and Storage Tips:
Consider preparing a batch of turkey and avocado wraps ahead of time and storing individual portions in airtight containers in the refrigerator for quick and convenient meals throughout the week. Add avocado just before serving to prevent browning.

By following these guidelines and incorporating turkey and avocado wraps into your diet, you can enjoy a delicious and nutritious meal that supports your health and well-being on the Blood Type O Diet.

Quinoa and Black Bean Salad

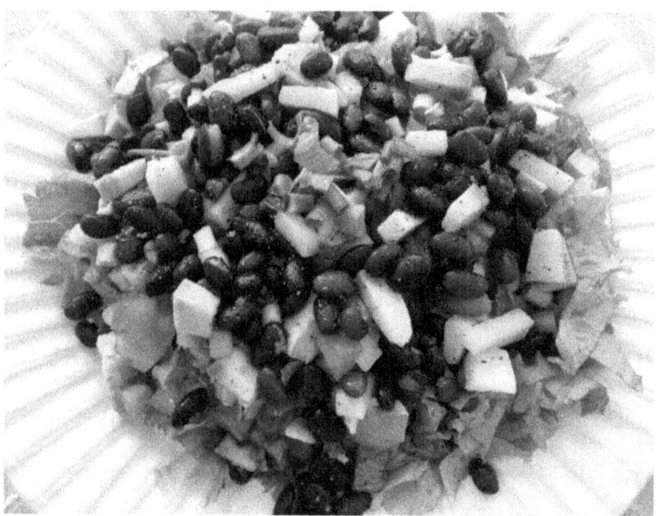

Quinoa and black bean salad is a nutritious and flavorful dish that is perfectly suited for individuals following the Blood Type O Diet. In this chapter, we explore how to create a delicious salad using blood type O-friendly ingredients.

1. Incorporating Blood Type O-Friendly Protein:

Black beans serve as the primary source of protein in this salad. They are rich in protein, fiber, and essential nutrients, making them an excellent choice for blood type O individuals. Black beans also provide a hearty texture and satisfying taste to the salad.

2. Using Blood Type O-Friendly Grains:

Quinoa is used as the grain base for this salad. It is a gluten-free pseudo-grain that is high in protein, fiber, and various vitamins and minerals. Quinoa adds a nutty flavor and fluffy texture to the salad while providing essential nutrients to support overall health and well-being.

3. Incorporating Blood Type O-Friendly Vegetables:

Add a variety of vegetables to your quinoa and black bean salad to increase fiber, vitamins, and minerals. Suitable options for blood type O individuals include bell peppers, tomatoes, red onions, corn, and cilantro. These vegetables add color, texture, and nutritional value to the salad.

4. Including Healthy Fats:

Incorporate avocado slices into your salad to add healthy fats, creaminess, and flavor. Avocado is rich in monounsaturated fats, which are beneficial for heart health and satiety. It also provides essential nutrients such as potassium, vitamin K, and folate.

5. Balancing Flavors and Textures:

Balance the flavors and textures of your quinoa and black bean salad by incorporating ingredients such as lime juice, olive oil, garlic, cumin, and chili powder. These seasonings add depth and complexity to the salad, enhancing its overall taste and appeal.

6. Customizing to Suit Individual Preferences:

Quinoa and black bean salad is highly customizable, allowing individuals to tailor ingredients and flavors to their liking. Experiment with different combinations of vegetables, herbs, and seasonings to create your perfect blood type O-friendly salad.

7. Adding Extra Protein and Texture:

Enhance the protein content and texture of your salad by adding additional blood type O-friendly ingredients such as grilled chicken, shrimp, or tofu. These additions provide extra satiety and nutritional value, making the salad more satisfying as a main dish.

8. Pairing with Blood Type O-Friendly Sides:

Serve your quinoa and black bean salad with blood type O-friendly sides such as mixed greens, sliced fruit, or whole grain bread. These options complement the flavors of the salad and provide additional nutrients and fiber.

9. Enjoying Mindfully:

Sit down and enjoy your quinoa and black bean salad mindfully, taking time to savor each bite and appreciate the nourishment it provides. Chew slowly, and listen to your body's hunger and fullness cues to promote digestion and satisfaction.

10. Meal Prep and Storage Tips:
Consider preparing a batch of quinoa and black bean salad ahead of time and storing individual portions in airtight containers in the refrigerator for quick and convenient meals throughout the week. Add avocado just before serving to prevent browning.

By following these guidelines and incorporating quinoa and black bean salad into your diet, you can enjoy a delicious and nutritious meal that supports your health and well-being on the Blood Type O Diet.

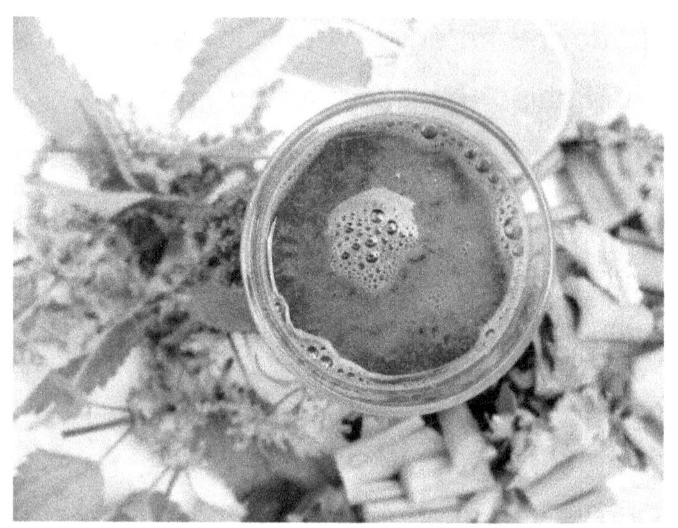

Chapter Four: Dinner Delights

Beef Stir-Fry with Broccoli and Bell Peppers

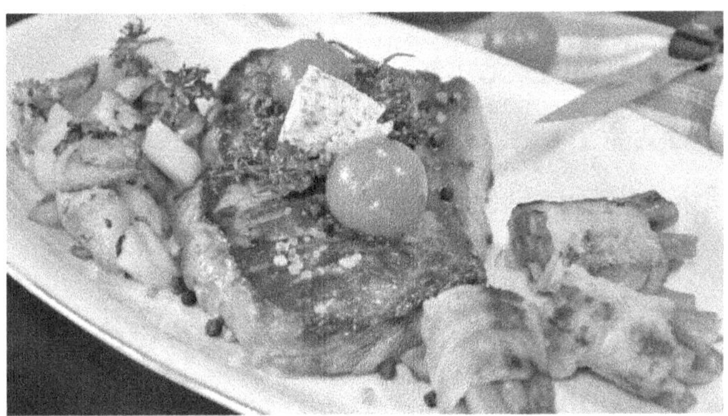

Beef stir-fry with broccoli and bell peppers is a flavorful and nutrient-rich dish that is well-suited for individuals following the Blood Type O Diet. In this chapter, we explore how to create a delicious stir-fry using blood type O-friendly ingredients.

1. Choosing Blood Type O-Friendly Protein:

Select lean beef cuts such as sirloin or flank steak as the protein source for your stir-fry. Beef is rich in high-quality protein, iron, and essential nutrients, making it an excellent choice for blood type O individuals. Opt for grass-fed or organic beef whenever possible for the highest quality and nutritional value.

2. Incorporating Blood Type O-Friendly Vegetables:

Add a variety of vegetables to your stir-fry to increase fiber, vitamins, and minerals. Suitable options for blood type O individuals include broccoli, bell peppers, onions, mushrooms, and snap peas. These vegetables add color, texture, and nutritional value to the dish.

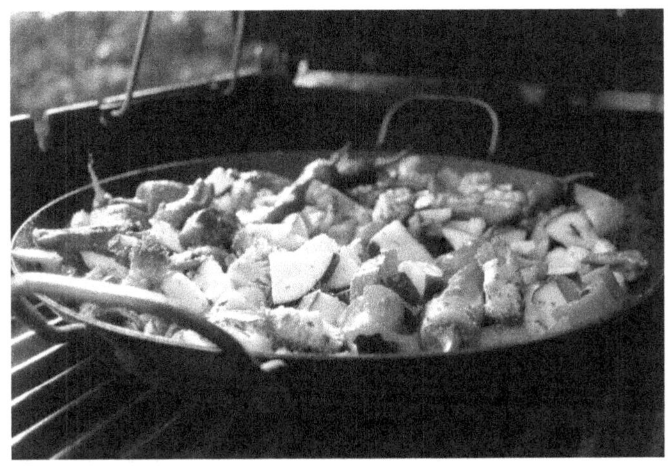

3. Using Blood Type O-Friendly Sauce:

Prepare a homemade stir-fry sauce using blood type O-friendly ingredients such as tamari or coconut aminos, garlic, ginger, and a touch of honey or maple syrup for sweetness. This sauce adds flavor and depth to the stir-fry without the need for added sugars or artificial ingredients.

4. Balancing Flavors and Textures:

Balance the flavors and textures of your beef stir-fry by incorporating ingredients such as fresh ginger, garlic, sesame oil, and red pepper flakes. These seasonings add complexity and depth to the dish, enhancing its overall taste and appeal.

5. Cooking Method:

Stir-frying is a quick and efficient cooking method that helps to preserve the nutrients and flavors of the ingredients. Use a wok or large skillet over high heat to cook the beef and vegetables quickly, ensuring they remain crisp and tender.

6. Pairing with Blood Type O-Friendly Sides:

Serve your beef stir-fry with blood type O-friendly sides such as brown rice, quinoa, or cauliflower rice. These options complement the flavors of the stir-fry and provide additional nutrients and fiber.

7. Adding Extra Nutrients:

Enhance the nutritional content of your stir-fry by adding additional blood type O-friendly ingredients such as sliced carrots, water chestnuts, or snow peas. These additions provide extra vitamins, minerals, and antioxidants to the dish.

8. Customizing to Suit Individual Preferences:

Beef stir-fry with broccoli and bell peppers is highly customizable, allowing individuals to tailor ingredients and flavors to their liking. Experiment with different combinations of vegetables, proteins, and seasonings to create your perfect blood type O-friendly stir-fry.

9. Enjoying Mindfully:

Sit down and enjoy your beef stir-fry with broccoli and bell peppers mindfully, taking time to savor each bite and appreciate the nourishment it provides. Chew slowly, and listen to your body's hunger and fullness cues to promote digestion and satisfaction.

10. Meal Prep and Storage Tips:

Consider preparing a batch of beef stir-fry ahead of time and storing individual portions in airtight containers in the refrigerator for quick and convenient meals throughout the week. Reheat leftovers in a skillet or microwave until heated through.

By following these guidelines and incorporating beef stir-fry with broccoli and bell peppers into your diet, you can enjoy a delicious and nutritious meal that supports your health and well-being on the Blood Type O Diet.

Salmon with Lemon and Dill

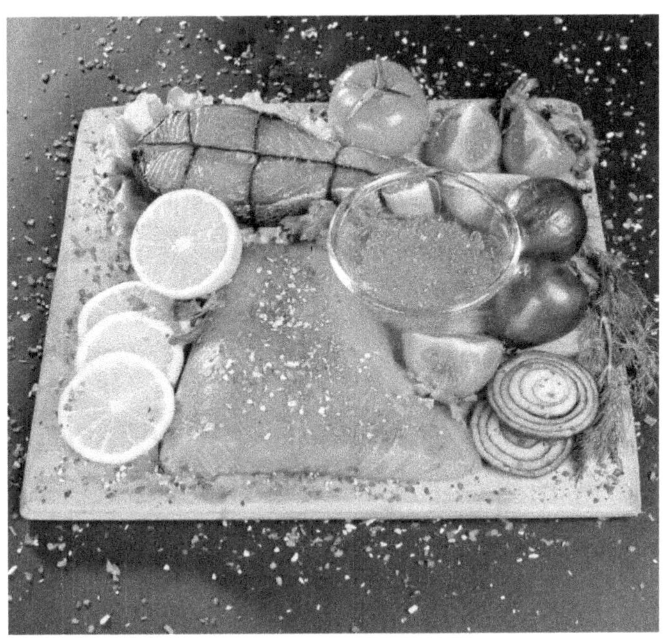

Salmon with lemon and dill is a delicious and nutritious dish that is perfectly suited for individuals following the Blood Type O Diet. In this chapter, we explore how to create a flavorful salmon dish using blood type O-friendly ingredients.

1. Choosing Blood Type O-Friendly Protein:

Select wild-caught salmon fillets as the protein source for your dish. Salmon is rich in omega-3 fatty acids, high-quality protein, and essential nutrients, making it an excellent choice for blood type O individuals. Opt for wild-caught salmon over farmed varieties for the highest nutritional value.

2. Incorporating Blood Type O-Friendly Herbs and Citrus:

Add fresh dill and lemon to your salmon dish to enhance its flavor and aroma. Dill provides a delicate, aromatic flavor that complements the richness of the salmon, while lemon adds brightness and acidity. These ingredients are compatible with the Blood Type O Diet and contribute to the overall deliciousness of the dish.

3. Using Healthy Cooking Methods:

Prepare your salmon using healthy cooking methods such as baking, grilling, or broiling. These methods help to preserve the nutrients and natural flavors of the fish without the need for excessive added fats or oils.

4. Balancing Flavors and Textures:

Balance the flavors and textures of your salmon dish by incorporating ingredients such as garlic, olive oil, salt, and pepper. These seasonings add depth and complexity to the dish, enhancing its overall taste and appeal.

5. Pairing with Blood Type O-Friendly Sides:

Serve your salmon with lemon and dill with blood type O-friendly sides such as steamed vegetables, roasted potatoes, or a mixed green salad. These options complement the flavors of the salmon and provide additional nutrients and fiber.

6. Adding Extra Nutrients:

Enhance the nutritional content of your salmon dish by adding additional blood type O-friendly ingredients such as asparagus, cherry tomatoes, or artichokes. These additions provide extra vitamins, minerals, and antioxidants to the dish.

7. Customizing to Suit Individual Preferences:

Salmon with lemon and dill is highly customizable, allowing individuals to tailor ingredients and flavors to their liking. Experiment with different combinations of herbs, citrus, and seasonings to create your perfect blood type O-friendly salmon dish.

8. Enjoying Mindfully:

Sit down and enjoy your salmon with lemon and dill mindfully, taking time to savor each bite and appreciate the nourishment it provides. Chew slowly, and listen to your body's hunger and fullness cues to promote digestion and satisfaction.

9. Meal Prep and Storage Tips:

Consider preparing a batch of salmon with lemon and dill ahead of time and storing individual portions in airtight containers in the refrigerator for quick and convenient meals throughout the week. Reheat leftovers gently to prevent overcooking.

10. Health Benefits of Salmon:

Salmon is not only delicious but also offers numerous health benefits, including support for heart health, brain function, and inflammation reduction due to its high omega-3 fatty acid content. Incorporating salmon into your diet regularly can contribute to overall well-being, making it an ideal choice for blood type O individuals.

By following these guidelines and incorporating salmon with lemon and dill into your diet, you can enjoy a flavorful and nutritious meal that supports your health and well-being on the Blood Type O Diet.

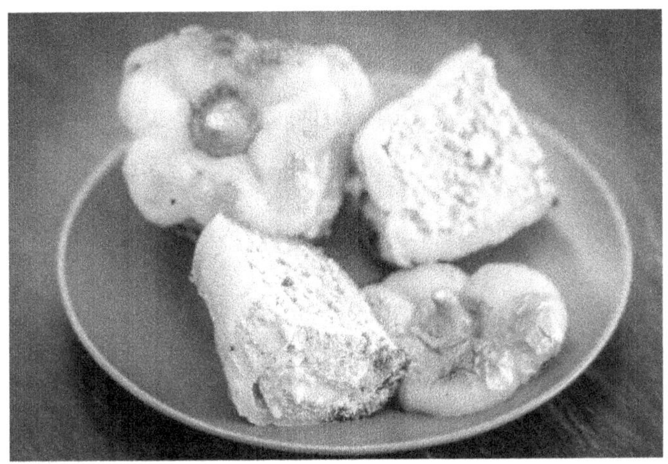

Stuffed bell peppers with ground turkey is a delicious and nutritious dish that is ideal for individuals following the Blood Type O Diet. In this chapter, we explore how to create a flavorful and protein-rich meal using blood type O-friendly ingredients.

1. Choosing Blood Type O-Friendly Protein:

Select lean ground turkey as the protein source for your stuffed bell peppers. Ground turkey is a lean alternative to beef, providing high-quality protein while being lower in fat. Opt for organic or free-range ground turkey for the best quality and nutritional value.

2. Incorporating Blood Type O-Friendly Vegetables:

Add a variety of vegetables to your stuffed bell peppers to increase fiber, vitamins, and minerals. Suitable options for blood type O individuals include onions, garlic, tomatoes, spinach, and mushrooms. These vegetables add flavor, texture, and nutritional value to the dish.

3. Using Blood Type O-Friendly Grains:

Incorporate cooked brown rice or quinoa into your stuffing mixture to add texture and nutritional value. These whole grains are compatible with the Blood Type O Diet and provide additional fiber, vitamins, and minerals.

4. Balancing Flavors and Seasonings:

Balance the flavors of your stuffed bell peppers by incorporating herbs, spices, and seasonings such as garlic, basil, oregano, and paprika. These seasonings add depth and complexity to the dish, enhancing its overall taste and appeal.

5. Choosing Blood Type O-Friendly Sauce:

Prepare a homemade tomato sauce using blood type O-friendly ingredients such as crushed tomatoes, garlic, olive oil, and herbs. This sauce adds moisture and flavor to the stuffed bell peppers without the need for added sugars or artificial ingredients.

6. Pairing with Blood Type O-Friendly Sides:

Serve your stuffed bell peppers with a side of mixed greens or a simple salad dressed with olive oil and lemon juice. These options complement the flavors of the peppers and provide additional nutrients and fiber.

7. Adding Extra Nutrients:

Enhance the nutritional content of your stuffed bell peppers by adding additional blood type O-friendly ingredients such as diced zucchini, black beans, or corn. These additions provide extra vitamins, minerals, and antioxidants to the dish.

8. Customizing to Suit Individual Preferences:

Stuffed bell peppers with ground turkey are highly customizable, allowing individuals to tailor ingredients and flavors to their liking. Experiment with different combinations of vegetables, grains, and seasonings to create your perfect blood type O-friendly stuffed peppers.

9. Enjoying Mindfully:

Sit down and enjoy your stuffed bell peppers with ground turkey mindfully, taking time to savor each bite and appreciate the nourishment it provides. Chew slowly, and listen to your body's hunger and fullness cues to promote digestion and satisfaction.

10. Meal Prep and Storage Tips:

Consider preparing a batch of stuffed bell peppers ahead of time and storing individual portions in airtight containers in the refrigerator or freezer for quick and convenient meals throughout the week. Reheat leftovers gently to preserve their texture and flavor.

By following these guidelines and incorporating stuffed bell peppers with ground turkey into your diet, you can enjoy a delicious and nutritious meal that supports your health and well-being on the Blood Type O Diet.

Chapter Five: Snacks and Appetizers

Crunchy Kale Chips

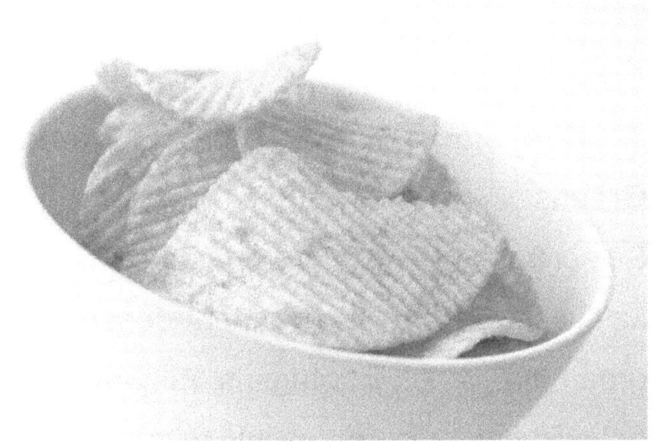

Crunchy kale chips are a nutritious and delicious snack option that perfectly aligns with the Blood Type O Diet. In this chapter, we explore how to create homemade kale chips using blood type O-friendly ingredients.

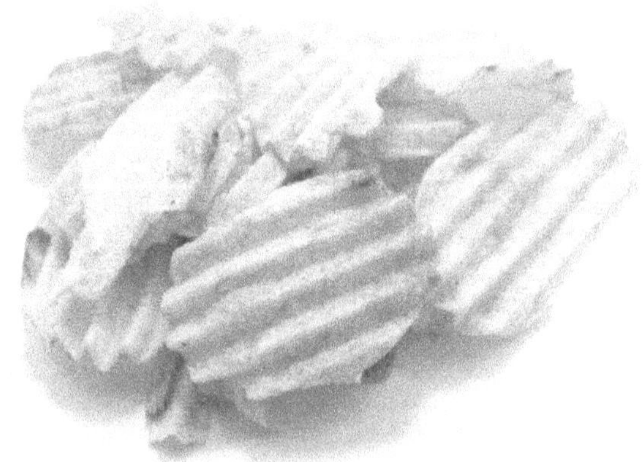

1. Choosing Blood Type O-Friendly Greens:

Select fresh kale leaves as the base for your kale chips. Kale is a nutrient-dense leafy green that is rich in vitamins, minerals, and antioxidants. It is compatible with the Blood Type O Diet and provides essential nutrients to support overall health and well-being.

2. Using Healthy Cooking Oil:

Coat the kale leaves lightly with blood type O-friendly cooking oil such as olive oil or avocado oil. These oils provide healthy fats and help to crisp up the kale chips during baking. Avoid using vegetable oils or other refined oils that may not be as beneficial for blood type O individuals.

3. Seasoning with Blood Type O-Friendly Herbs and Spices:

Season your kale chips with blood type O-friendly herbs, spices, and seasonings such as garlic powder, onion powder, paprika, or nutritional yeast. These ingredients add flavor and depth to the chips without the need for added sugars or artificial flavorings.

4. Adding Crunch with Nuts or Seeds:

Enhance the texture and nutritional value of your kale chips by sprinkling them with blood type O-friendly nuts or seeds such as sesame seeds, pumpkin seeds, or sunflower seeds before baking. These additions add crunch and protein to the chips, making them even more satisfying as a snack.

5. Baking Method:

Preheat your oven to a low temperature (around 300°F or 150°C) and spread the seasoned kale leaves in a single layer on a baking sheet lined with parchment paper. Bake the kale chips for 10-15 minutes, or until they are crispy and lightly golden brown. Be sure to watch them closely to prevent burning.

6. Pairing with Blood Type O-Friendly Dips:

Serve your crunchy kale chips with blood type O-friendly dips such as guacamole, hummus, or tzatziki. These options complement the flavor of the chips and provide additional nutrients and flavor to the snack.

7. Customizing to Suit Individual Preferences:

Crunchy kale chips are highly customizable, allowing individuals to tailor ingredients and flavors to their liking. Experiment with different seasonings, nuts, seeds, and dips to create your perfect blood type O-friendly snack.

8. Enjoying Mindfully:

Enjoy your crunchy kale chips mindfully, taking time to savor each crispy bite and appreciate the nourishment they provide. Kale chips are a satisfying and guilt-free snack option that can be enjoyed any time of day.

9. Portion Control:

While kale chips are a nutritious snack, it's essential to practice portion control, especially if you're watching your calorie intake or trying to manage your weight. Enjoy them in moderation as part of a balanced diet.

10. Storage Tips:

Store any leftover kale chips in an airtight container at room temperature for up to a few days. Be sure to keep them in a cool, dry place to maintain their crispiness.

By following these guidelines and incorporating crunchy kale chips into your diet, you can enjoy a flavorful and nutritious snack that supports your health and well-being on the Blood Type O Diet.

Hummus and Veggie Platter

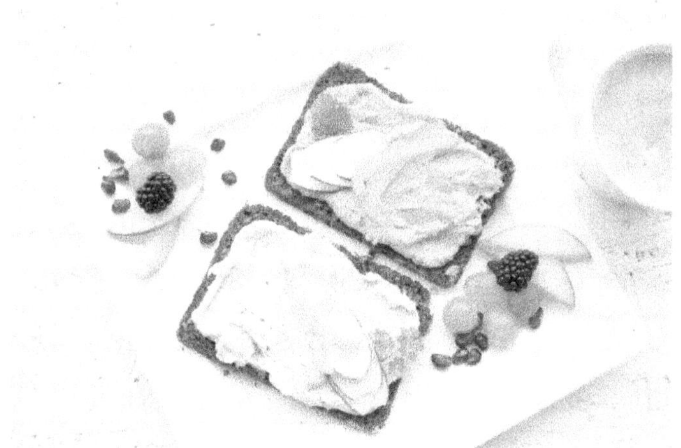

A hummus and veggie platter is a nutritious and satisfying snack or appetizer option that is perfectly suited for individuals following the Blood Type O Diet. In this chapter, we explore how to create a delicious platter using blood type O-friendly ingredients.

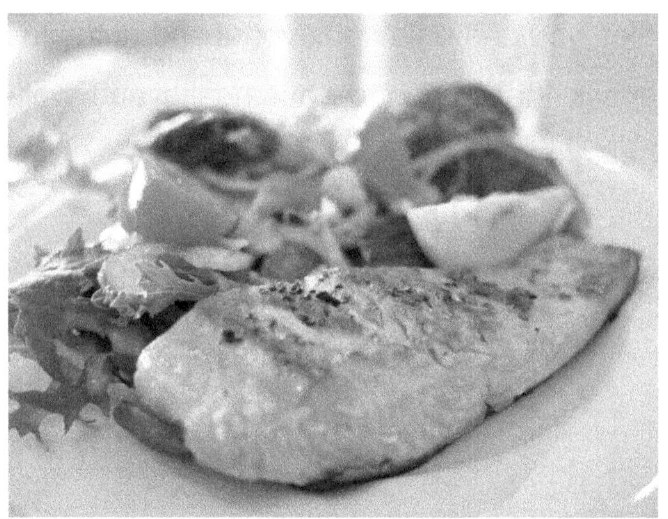

1. Choosing Blood Type O-Friendly Dip:

Select hummus as the main dip for your veggie platter. Hummus is made from chickpeas, which are a great source of protein, fiber, and essential nutrients. Opt for homemade or store-bought hummus without added sugars or artificial ingredients.

2. Incorporating Blood Type O-Friendly Vegetables:

Add a variety of raw vegetables to your platter to increase fiber, vitamins, and minerals. Suitable options for blood type O individuals include carrot sticks, cucumber slices, bell pepper strips, cherry tomatoes, and snap peas. These vegetables add color, texture, and nutritional value to the platter.

3. Including Blood Type O-Friendly Extras:

Enhance the flavor and nutritional content of your platter by incorporating additional blood type O-friendly extras such as olives, pickles, or roasted nuts. These additions provide extra flavor, texture, and nutrients to the platter.

4. Balancing Flavors and Textures:

Balance the flavors and textures of your hummus and veggie platter by incorporating a variety of ingredients with different tastes and mouthfeels. Consider adding crunchy vegetables, creamy hummus, tangy olives, and savory nuts to create a well-rounded and satisfying snack.

5. Pairing with Blood Type O-Friendly Sides:

Serve your hummus and veggie platter with blood type O-friendly sides such as whole grain crackers, pita bread, or rice cakes. These options complement the flavors of the vegetables and hummus and provide additional nutrients and fiber.

6. Customizing to Suit Individual Preferences:

A hummus and veggie platter is highly customizable, allowing individuals to tailor ingredients and flavors to their liking. Experiment with different combinations of vegetables, dips, and extras to create your perfect blood type O-friendly platter.

7. Portion Control:

While hummus and vegetables are nutritious, it's essential to practice portion control, especially if you're watching your calorie intake or trying to manage your weight. Enjoy your platter in moderation as part of a balanced diet.

8. Enjoying Mindfully:

Sit down and enjoy your hummus and veggie platter mindfully, taking time to savor each bite and appreciate the nourishment it provides. Chew slowly, and listen to your body's hunger and fullness cues to promote digestion and satisfaction.

9. Meal Prep and Storage Tips:

Prepare your hummus and chop your vegetables ahead of time for quick and convenient snacking throughout the week. Store any leftovers in airtight containers in the refrigerator to keep them fresh.

By following these guidelines and incorporating a hummus and veggie platter into your diet, you can enjoy a delicious and nutritious snack that supports your health and well-being on the Blood Type O Diet.

Spicy Edamame

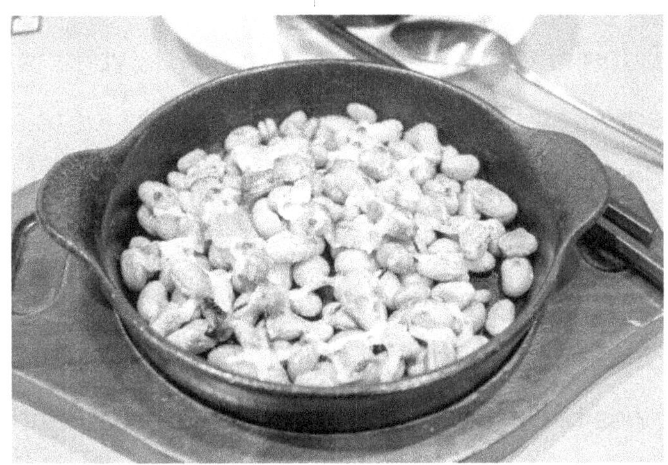

Spicy edamame is a flavorful and nutritious snack option that is well-suited for individuals following the Blood Type O Diet. In this chapter, we explore how to create a delicious and spicy edamame dish using blood type O-friendly ingredients.

1. Choosing Blood Type O-Friendly Protein:

Edamame, which are young soybeans, serve as the primary protein source for this dish. Edamame is rich in protein, fiber, and essential nutrients, making it an excellent choice for blood type O individuals. Opt for organic or non-GMO edamame whenever possible for the highest quality and nutritional value.

2. Seasoning with Blood Type O-Friendly Spices:

Season your edamame with blood type O-friendly spices and seasonings to add flavor and heat. Suitable options include crushed red pepper flakes, garlic powder, onion powder, paprika, and cayenne pepper. These spices add depth and complexity to the dish without the need for added sugars or artificial flavorings.

3. Adding Healthy Fats:

Drizzle your spicy edamame with blood type O-friendly fats such as olive oil or sesame oil. These oils provide healthy fats and help to coat the edamame evenly, enhancing the flavor and texture of the dish.

4. Balancing Flavors and Textures:

Balance the flavors and textures of your spicy edamame by incorporating ingredients such as soy sauce or tamari, rice vinegar, and a touch of sweetness from honey or maple syrup. These ingredients create a savory, umami-rich sauce that complements the heat of the spices.

5. Cooking Method:

Cook your edamame by boiling them in salted water for a few minutes until they are tender but still firm. Drain the edamame and then toss them in the spicy seasoning mixture until they are evenly coated.

6. Pairing with Blood Type O-Friendly Sides:

Serve your spicy edamame with blood type O-friendly sides such as brown rice, quinoa, or a side of steamed vegetables. These options complement the flavors of the edamame and provide additional nutrients and fiber.

7. Customizing to Suit Individual Preferences:

Spicy edamame is highly customizable, allowing individuals to tailor ingredients and flavors to their liking. Experiment with different combinations of spices, seasonings, and sauces to create your perfect blood type O-friendly dish.

8. Enjoying Mindfully:

Sit down and enjoy your spicy edamame mindfully, taking time to savor each bite and appreciate the nourishment it provides. Edamame is a satisfying and nutritious snack that can be enjoyed any time of day.

9. Portion Control:

While edamame is a nutritious snack, it's essential to practice portion control, especially if you're watching your calorie intake or trying to manage your weight. Enjoy your spicy edamame in moderation as part of a balanced diet.

10. Meal Prep and Storage Tips:

Prepare a batch of spicy edamame ahead of time and store individual portions in airtight containers in the refrigerator for quick and convenient snacking throughout the week. Reheat leftovers gently to preserve their texture and flavor.

By following these guidelines and incorporating spicy edamame into your diet, you can enjoy a flavorful and nutritious snack that supports your health and well-being on the Blood Type O Diet.

Chapter Six: Soups and Stews

Classic Chicken Soup

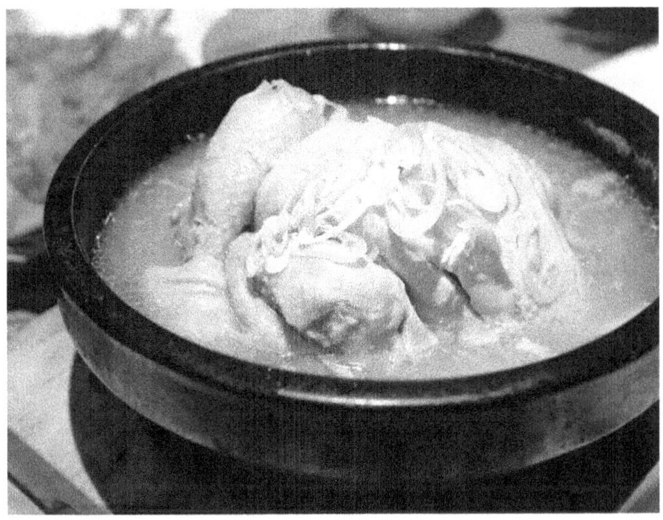

Classic chicken soup is a comforting and nutritious dish that is suitable for individuals following the Blood Type O Diet. In this chapter, we explore how to create a delicious and hearty chicken soup using blood type O-friendly ingredients.

1. Choosing Blood Type O-Friendly Protein:

Select lean chicken breast or thigh meat as the protein source for your soup. Chicken is a versatile protein that is rich in essential nutrients such as protein, vitamins, and minerals. Opt for organic or free-range chicken whenever possible for the best quality and nutritional value.

2. Incorporating Blood Type O-Friendly Vegetables:

Add a variety of vegetables to your chicken soup to increase fiber, vitamins, and minerals. Suitable options for blood type O individuals include onions, carrots, celery, garlic, and leafy greens such as kale or spinach. These vegetables add flavor, texture, and nutritional value to the soup.

3. Using Blood Type O-Friendly Herbs and Spices:

Season your chicken soup with blood type O-friendly herbs and spices such as thyme, parsley, bay leaves, and black pepper. These seasonings add depth and complexity to the soup without the need for added sugars or artificial flavorings.

4. Adding Healthy Fats:

Drizzle your chicken soup with blood type O-friendly fats such as olive oil or avocado oil. These oils provide healthy fats and help to enhance the flavor and richness of the soup.

5. Balancing Flavors and Textures:

Balance the flavors and textures of your chicken soup by incorporating ingredients such as chicken broth, lemon juice, and a touch of sweetness from carrots or tomatoes. These ingredients create a savory and satisfying broth that complements the tender chicken and vegetables.

6. Cooking Method:

Cook your chicken soup slowly over low heat to allow the flavors to meld together and the chicken to become tender. Simmer the soup for at least 30 minutes to an hour, stirring occasionally to prevent sticking.

7. Pairing with Blood Type O-Friendly Sides:

Serve your classic chicken soup with blood type O-friendly sides such as whole grain bread, brown rice, or quinoa. These options complement the flavors of the soup and provide additional nutrients and fiber.

8. Customizing to Suit Individual Preferences:

Classic chicken soup is highly customizable, allowing individuals to tailor ingredients and flavors to their liking. Experiment with different combinations of vegetables, herbs, and spices to create your perfect blood type O-friendly soup.

9. Enjoying Mindfully:

Sit down and enjoy your classic chicken soup mindfully, taking time to savor each spoonful and appreciate the nourishment it provides. Chicken soup is a comforting and satisfying meal that can be enjoyed any time of day.

10. Meal Prep and Storage Tips:

Prepare a batch of classic chicken soup ahead of time and store individual portions in airtight containers in the refrigerator or freezer for quick and convenient meals throughout the week. Reheat leftovers gently to preserve their flavor and texture.

By following these guidelines and incorporating classic chicken soup into your diet, you can enjoy a flavorful and nutritious meal that supports your health and well-being on the Blood Type O Diet.

Lentil and Vegetable Stew

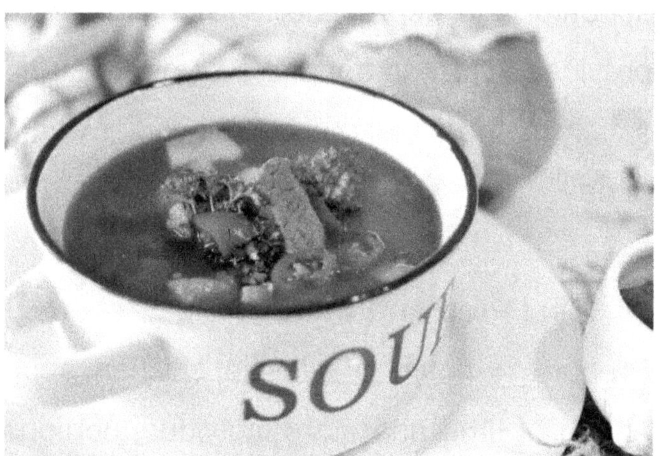

Lentil and vegetable stew is a hearty and nutritious dish that is perfect for individuals following the Blood Type O Diet. In this chapter, we explore how to create a flavorful stew using blood type O-friendly ingredients.

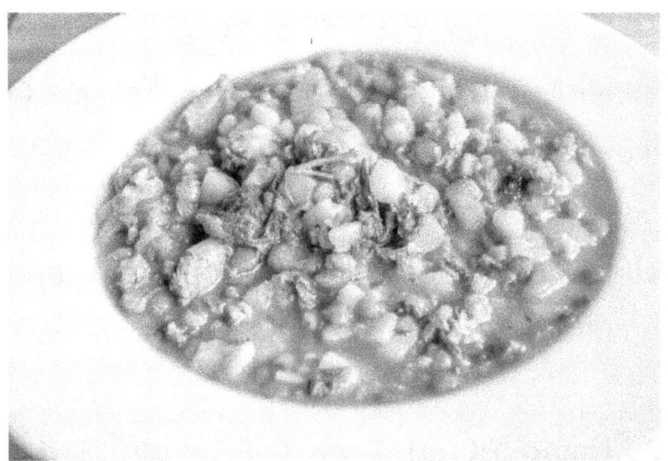

1. Choosing Blood Type O-Friendly Protein:

Lentils serve as the primary protein source for this stew. Lentils are rich in protein, fiber, and essential nutrients, making them an excellent choice for blood type O individuals. Opt for green or brown lentils, which hold their shape well during cooking and provide a hearty texture to the stew.

2. Incorporating Blood Type O-Friendly Vegetables:

Add a variety of vegetables to your lentil stew to increase fiber, vitamins, and minerals. Suitable options for blood type O individuals include onions, carrots, celery, bell peppers, and tomatoes. These vegetables add flavor, texture, and nutritional value to the stew.

3. Using Blood Type O-Friendly Herbs and Spices:

Season your lentil stew with blood type O-friendly herbs and spices such as garlic, thyme, rosemary, cumin, and smoked paprika. These seasonings add depth and complexity to the stew without the need for added sugars or artificial flavorings.

4. Adding Healthy Fats:

Drizzle your lentil stew with blood type O-friendly fats such as olive oil or avocado oil. These oils provide healthy fats and help to enhance the flavor and richness of the stew.

5. Balancing Flavors and Textures:

Balance the flavors and textures of your lentil stew by incorporating ingredients such as vegetable broth, diced tomatoes, and a touch of sweetness from carrots or sweet potatoes. These ingredients create a savory and satisfying broth that complements the hearty lentils and vegetables.

6. Cooking Method:

Cook your lentil stew slowly over low heat to allow the flavors to meld together and the lentils to become tender. Simmer the stew for at least 45 minutes to an hour, stirring occasionally to prevent sticking.

7. Pairing with Blood Type O-Friendly Sides:

Serve your lentil and vegetable stew with blood type O-friendly sides such as whole grain bread, brown rice, or a side salad. These options complement the flavors of the stew and provide additional nutrients and fiber.

8. Customizing to Suit Individual Preferences:

Lentil and vegetable stew is highly customizable, allowing individuals to tailor ingredients and flavors to their liking. Experiment with different combinations of vegetables, herbs, and spices to create your perfect blood type O-friendly stew.

9. Enjoying Mindfully:

Sit down and enjoy your lentil and vegetable stew mindfully, taking time to savor each spoonful and appreciate the nourishment it provides. Lentil stew is a comforting and satisfying meal that can be enjoyed any time of day.

10. Meal Prep and Storage Tips:

Prepare a batch of lentil and vegetable stew ahead of time and store individual portions in airtight containers in the refrigerator or freezer for quick and convenient meals throughout the week. Reheat leftovers gently to preserve their flavor and texture.

By following these guidelines and incorporating lentil and vegetable stew into your diet, you can enjoy a flavorful and nutritious meal that supports your health and well-being on the Blood Type O Diet.

Tomato Basil Soup with Chickpeas

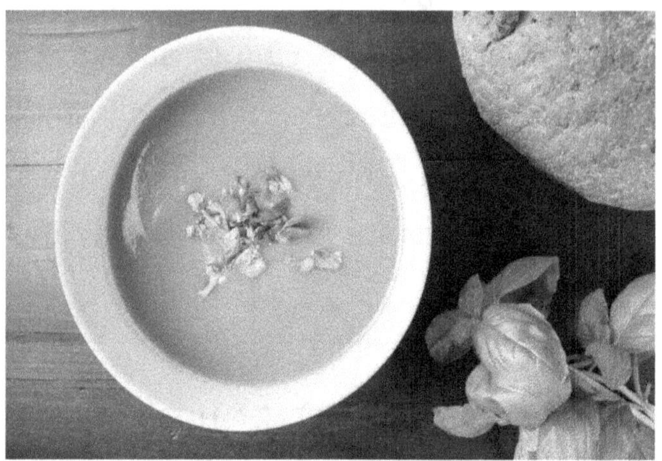

Tomato basil soup with chickpeas is a delicious and nutritious dish that aligns well with the Blood Type O Diet. In this chapter, we explore how to create a flavorful soup using blood type O-friendly ingredients.

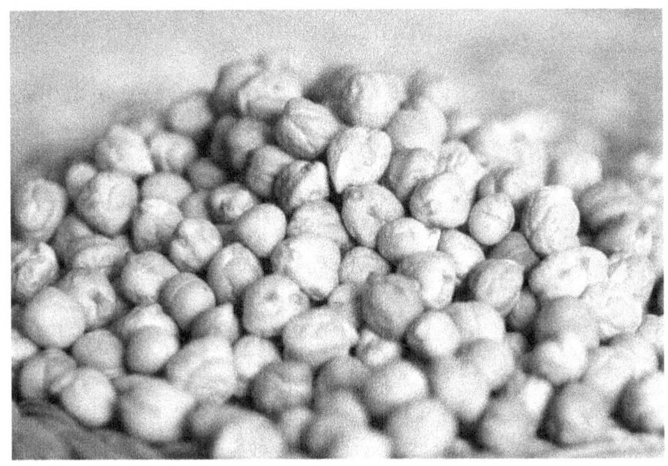

1. Choosing Blood Type O-Friendly Ingredients:

Select fresh tomatoes, basil, and chickpeas as the main ingredients for your soup. Tomatoes are rich in antioxidants like lycopene and vitamin C, while basil adds a fragrant and aromatic flavor. Chickpeas provide plant-based protein and fiber, making them a filling addition to the soup.

2. Incorporating Blood Type O-Friendly Herbs and Spices:

Season your tomato basil soup with blood type O-friendly herbs and spices such as garlic, onion powder, oregano, and black pepper. These seasonings enhance the flavor of the soup without the need for added salt or artificial ingredients.

3. Adding Healthy Fats:

Drizzle your soup with blood type O-friendly fats such as extra virgin olive oil. Olive oil not only adds richness to the soup but also provides heart-healthy monounsaturated fats.

4. Balancing Flavors and Textures:

Balance the flavors and textures of your tomato basil soup by incorporating ingredients such as vegetable broth, diced tomatoes, and cooked chickpeas. These ingredients create a savory and satisfying soup with a rich, creamy texture.

5. Cooking Method:

Simmer your soup over low heat to allow the flavors to meld together and the chickpeas to become tender. Stir occasionally to prevent sticking and ensure that the soup cooks evenly.

6. Pairing with Blood Type O-Friendly Sides:

Serve your tomato basil soup with chickpeas with blood type O-friendly sides such as whole grain bread, quinoa, or a side salad. These options complement the flavors of the soup and provide additional nutrients and fiber.

7. Customizing to Suit Individual Preferences:

Tomato basil soup with chickpeas is highly customizable, allowing individuals to tailor ingredients and flavors to their liking. Experiment with different combinations of herbs, spices, and vegetables to create your perfect blood type O-friendly soup.

8. Enjoying Mindfully:

Sit down and enjoy your tomato basil soup with chickpeas mindfully, taking time to savor each spoonful and appreciate the nourishment it provides. Soup can be a comforting and satisfying meal that can be enjoyed any time of day.

9. Portion Control:

While tomato basil soup with chickpeas is a nutritious option, it's important to practice portion control, especially if you're watching your calorie intake or trying to manage your weight. Enjoy your soup in moderation as part of a balanced diet.

10. Meal Prep and Storage Tips:

Prepare a batch of tomato basil soup with chickpeas ahead of time and store individual portions in airtight containers in the refrigerator or freezer for quick and convenient meals throughout the week. Reheat leftovers gently to preserve their flavor and texture.

By following these guidelines and incorporating tomato basil soup with chickpeas into your diet, you can enjoy a flavorful and nutritious meal that supports your health and well-being on the Blood Type O Diet.

Chapter Seven: Satisfying Sides

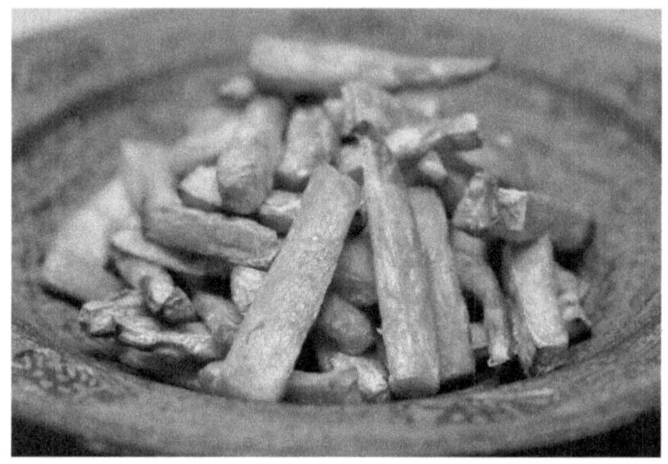

Roasted sweet potatoes are a delicious and nutritious side dish that fits well into the Blood Type O Diet. In this chapter, we explore how to create flavorful roasted sweet potatoes using blood type O-friendly ingredients.

1. Choosing Blood Type O-Friendly Ingredients:

Select fresh sweet potatoes as the main ingredient for your dish. Sweet potatoes are rich in vitamins, minerals, and fiber, making them an excellent choice for blood type O individuals. Opt for organic sweet potatoes whenever possible for the best quality and nutritional value.

2. Incorporating Blood Type O-Friendly Herbs and Spices:

Season your sweet potatoes with blood type O-friendly herbs and spices such as rosemary, thyme, paprika, garlic powder, or cinnamon. These seasonings add flavor and depth to the sweet potatoes without the need for added sugars or artificial flavorings.

3. Using Healthy Cooking Oil:

Coat your sweet potatoes lightly with blood type O-friendly cooking oil such as olive oil or avocado oil. These oils provide healthy fats and help to crisp up the sweet potatoes during roasting.

4. Balancing Flavors and Textures:

Balance the flavors and textures of your roasted sweet potatoes by incorporating ingredients such as sea salt, black pepper, and a touch of sweetness from maple syrup or honey. These ingredients enhance the natural sweetness of the sweet potatoes and create a delicious caramelized crust during roasting.

5. Cooking Method:

Roast your sweet potatoes in the oven at a moderate temperature (around 400°F or 200°C) until they are tender and golden brown, stirring occasionally to ensure even cooking. Roasting sweet potatoes helps to bring out their natural sweetness and enhances their flavor and texture.

6. Pairing with Blood Type O-Friendly Proteins:

Serve your roasted sweet potatoes with blood type O-friendly proteins such as grilled chicken, salmon, or tofu. These options complement the flavors of the sweet potatoes and provide additional nutrients and protein to the meal.

7. Customizing to Suit Individual Preferences:

Roasted sweet potatoes are highly customizable, allowing individuals to tailor ingredients and flavors to their liking. Experiment with different combinations of herbs, spices, and seasonings to create your perfect blood type O-friendly side dish.

8. Enjoying Mindfully:

Sit down and enjoy your roasted sweet potatoes mindfully, taking time to savor each bite and appreciate the nourishment they provide. Sweet potatoes are a satisfying and nutritious side dish that can be enjoyed any time of day.

9. Portion Control:

While sweet potatoes are nutritious, it's important to practice portion control, especially if you're watching your calorie intake or trying to manage your weight. Enjoy your roasted sweet potatoes in moderation as part of a balanced diet.

10. Meal Prep and Storage Tips:

Prepare a batch of roasted sweet potatoes ahead of time and store leftovers in an airtight container in the refrigerator for up to several days. Reheat them gently in the oven or microwave before serving to preserve their texture and flavor.

By following these guidelines and incorporating roasted sweet potatoes into your diet, you can enjoy a flavorful and nutritious side dish that supports your health and well-being on the Blood Type O Diet.

Garlic Sauteed Spinach

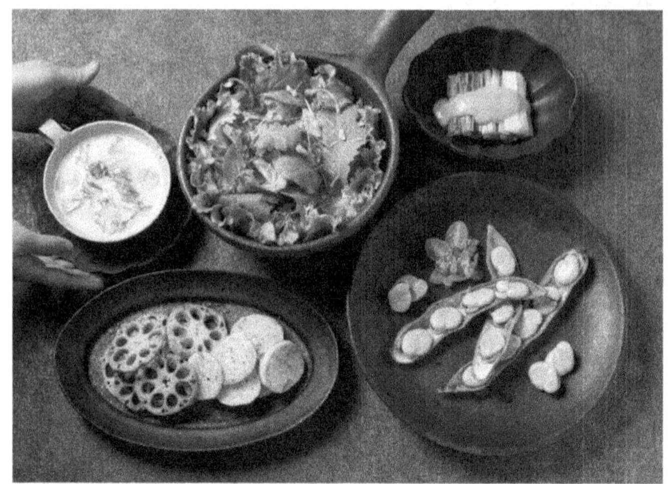

Garlic sautéed spinach is a delicious and nutrient-rich side dish that perfectly complements the Blood Type O Diet. In this chapter, we explore how to create flavorful garlic sautéed spinach using blood type O-friendly ingredients.

1. Choosing Blood Type O-Friendly Ingredients:

Select fresh spinach as the main ingredient for your dish. Spinach is a nutrient-dense leafy green that is rich in vitamins, minerals, and antioxidants, making it an excellent choice for blood type O individuals. Opt for organic spinach whenever possible for the best quality and nutritional value.

2. Incorporating Blood Type O-Friendly Herbs and Spices:

Season your spinach with blood type O-friendly herbs and spices such as garlic, onion powder, black pepper, and a touch of red pepper flakes for heat. These seasonings add flavor and depth to the spinach without the need for added salt or artificial flavorings.

3. Using Healthy Cooking Oil:

Sauté your spinach in blood type O-friendly cooking oil such as olive oil or avocado oil. These oils provide healthy fats and help to enhance the flavor of the spinach without adding unnecessary calories or unhealthy fats.

4. Balancing Flavors and Textures:

Balance the flavors and textures of your garlic sautéed spinach by incorporating ingredients such as minced garlic, lemon juice, and a pinch of nutmeg. These ingredients add complexity to the dish and enhance the natural sweetness of the spinach.

5. Cooking Method:

Sauté your spinach in a skillet over medium heat until it wilts down and becomes tender, stirring occasionally to ensure even cooking. Be careful not to overcook the spinach, as it can become mushy and lose its vibrant color and flavor.

6. Pairing with Blood Type O-Friendly Proteins:

Serve your garlic sautéed spinach with blood type O-friendly proteins such as grilled chicken, salmon, or tofu. These options complement the flavors of the spinach and provide additional nutrients and protein to the meal.

7. Customizing to Suit Individual Preferences:

Garlic sautéed spinach is highly customizable, allowing individuals to tailor ingredients and flavors to their liking. Experiment with different combinations of herbs, spices, and seasonings to create your perfect blood type O-friendly side dish.

8. Enjoying Mindfully:

Sit down and enjoy your garlic sautéed spinach mindfully, taking time to savor each bite and appreciate the nourishment it provides. Spinach is a versatile and nutritious vegetable that can be enjoyed as part of any meal.

9. Portion Control:

While spinach is nutritious, it's important to practice portion control, especially if you're watching your calorie intake or trying to manage your weight. Enjoy your garlic sautéed spinach in moderation as part of a balanced diet.

10. Meal Prep and Storage Tips:

Prepare a batch of garlic sautéed spinach ahead of time and store leftovers in an airtight container in the refrigerator for up to several days. Reheat them gently in a skillet or microwave before serving to preserve their texture and flavor.

By following these guidelines and incorporating garlic sautéed spinach into your diet, you can enjoy a flavorful and nutritious side dish that supports your health and well-being on the Blood Type O Diet.

Cauliflower Rice Pilaf

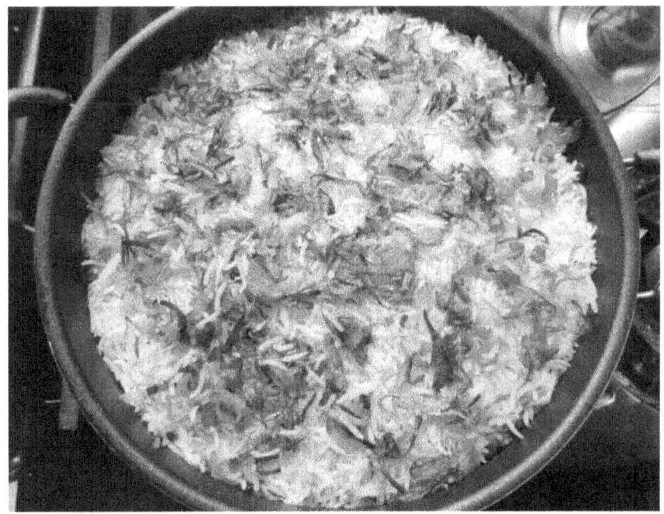

Cauliflower rice pilaf is a delicious and low-carb alternative to traditional rice pilaf that perfectly fits the Blood Type O Diet. In this chapter, we explore how to create a flavorful cauliflower rice pilaf using blood type O-friendly ingredients.

1. Choosing Blood Type O-Friendly Ingredients:

Select fresh cauliflower as the main ingredient for your pilaf. Cauliflower is a versatile vegetable that is low in carbohydrates and calories, making it an excellent choice for blood type O individuals. Opt for organic cauliflower whenever possible for the best quality and nutritional value.

2. Incorporating Blood Type O-Friendly Herbs and Spices:

Season your cauliflower rice pilaf with blood type O-friendly herbs and spices such as garlic, onion powder, turmeric, cumin, and paprika. These seasonings add flavor and depth to the pilaf without the need for added salt or artificial flavorings.

3. Adding Blood Type O-Friendly Vegetables:

Enhance the nutritional value of your cauliflower rice pilaf by incorporating blood type O-friendly vegetables such as onions, carrots, bell peppers, and peas. These vegetables add color, texture, and fiber to the pilaf, making it more satisfying and nutritious.

4. Using Healthy Cooking Oil:

Sauté your cauliflower rice pilaf in blood type O-friendly cooking oil such as olive oil or avocado oil. These oils provide healthy fats and help to enhance the flavor of the pilaf without adding unnecessary calories or unhealthy fats.

5. Balancing Flavors and Textures:

Balance the flavors and textures of your cauliflower rice pilaf by incorporating ingredients such as vegetable broth, lemon juice, and a touch of sweetness from raisins or dried cranberries. These ingredients create a savory and satisfying pilaf with a hint of sweetness.

6. Cooking Method:

Cook your cauliflower rice pilaf in a skillet over medium heat until the cauliflower is tender and the flavors have melded together, stirring occasionally to ensure even cooking. Be careful not to overcook the cauliflower, as it can become mushy and lose its texture.

7. Pairing with Blood Type O-Friendly Proteins:

Serve your cauliflower rice pilaf with blood type O-friendly proteins such as grilled chicken, shrimp, or tofu. These options complement the flavors of the pilaf and provide additional nutrients and protein to the meal.

8. Customizing to Suit Individual Preferences:

Cauliflower rice pilaf is highly customizable, allowing individuals to tailor ingredients and flavors to their liking. Experiment with different combinations of vegetables, herbs, and spices to create your perfect blood type O-friendly side dish.

9. Enjoying Mindfully:

Sit down and enjoy your cauliflower rice pilaf mindfully, taking time to savor each bite and appreciate the nourishment it provides. Cauliflower rice pilaf is a satisfying and flavorful dish that can be enjoyed as part of any meal.

10. Meal Prep and Storage Tips:

Prepare a batch of cauliflower rice pilaf ahead of time and store leftovers in an airtight container in the refrigerator for up to several days. Reheat them gently in a skillet or microwave before serving to preserve their texture and flavor.

By following these guidelines and incorporating cauliflower rice pilaf into your diet, you can enjoy a delicious and nutritious side dish that supports your health and well-being on the Blood Type O Diet.

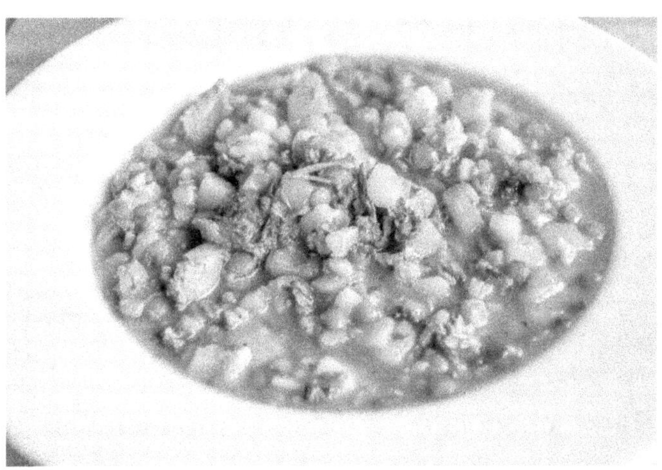

Chapter Eight: Dessert Indulgences

Dark Chocolate Avocado Mousse

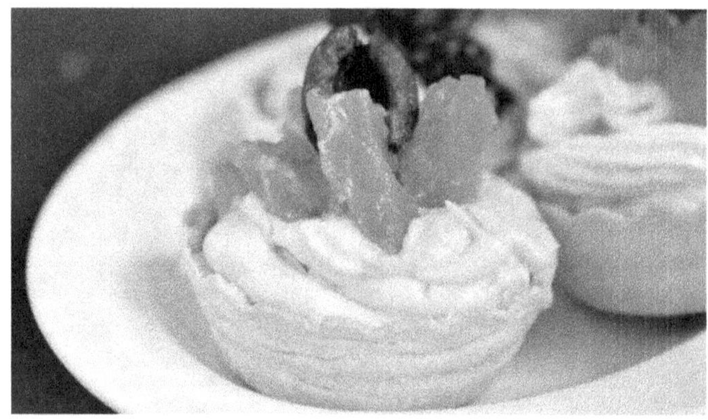

Dark chocolate avocado mousse is a decadent and satisfying dessert option that can be enjoyed by individuals following the Blood Type O Diet. In this chapter, we explore how to create a creamy and indulgent mousse using blood type O-friendly ingredients.

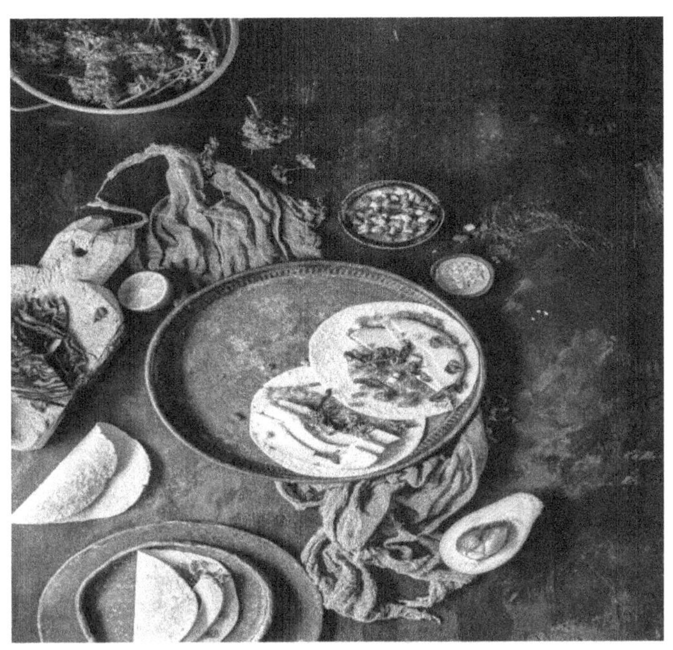

1. Choosing Blood Type O-Friendly Ingredients:

Select ripe avocados and high-quality dark chocolate as the main ingredients for your mousse. Avocados are rich in healthy fats and nutrients, while dark chocolate provides antioxidants and a rich, chocolatey flavor. Opt for dark chocolate with a cocoa content of at least 70% for the best flavor and health benefits.

2. Incorporating Blood Type O-Friendly Sweeteners:

Sweeten your mousse with blood type O-friendly sweeteners such as honey, maple syrup, or coconut sugar. These natural sweeteners add sweetness to the mousse without the need for refined sugars or artificial sweeteners.

3. Adding Flavor and Creaminess:

Enhance the flavor and creaminess of your mousse by incorporating ingredients such as vanilla extract, almond extract, or a splash of coconut milk. These additions add depth of flavor and help to achieve a smooth and velvety texture.

4. Balancing Flavors:

Balance the flavors of your dark chocolate avocado mousse by adding a pinch of sea salt or a splash of citrus juice such as lemon or orange. These ingredients help to enhance the richness of the chocolate and create a more complex flavor profile.

5. Preparation Method:

Blend together ripe avocados, melted dark chocolate, sweeteners, flavorings, and any additional ingredients until smooth and creamy. Adjust the sweetness and flavorings to taste, and chill the mousse in the refrigerator for at least an hour before serving to allow the flavors to meld together.

6. Serving Suggestions:

Serve your dark chocolate avocado mousse in individual dessert cups or bowls, garnished with a sprinkle of cocoa powder, grated dark chocolate, or fresh berries. This dessert can be enjoyed on its own or paired with a dollop of whipped coconut cream for added indulgence.

7. Portion Control:

While dark chocolate avocado mousse is a delicious treat, it's important to practice portion control, especially if you're watching your calorie intake or trying to manage your weight. Enjoy a small serving of mousse as an occasional indulgence rather than a regular part of your diet.

8. Meal Prep and Storage Tips:

Prepare your dark chocolate avocado mousse ahead of time and store leftovers in individual airtight containers in the refrigerator for up to a few days. Enjoy chilled straight from the fridge or allow to come to room temperature for a creamier texture.

By following these guidelines and incorporating dark chocolate avocado mousse into your diet, you can enjoy a rich and indulgent dessert that satisfies your sweet tooth while still supporting your health and well-being on the Blood Type O Diet.

Berry Almond Crumble

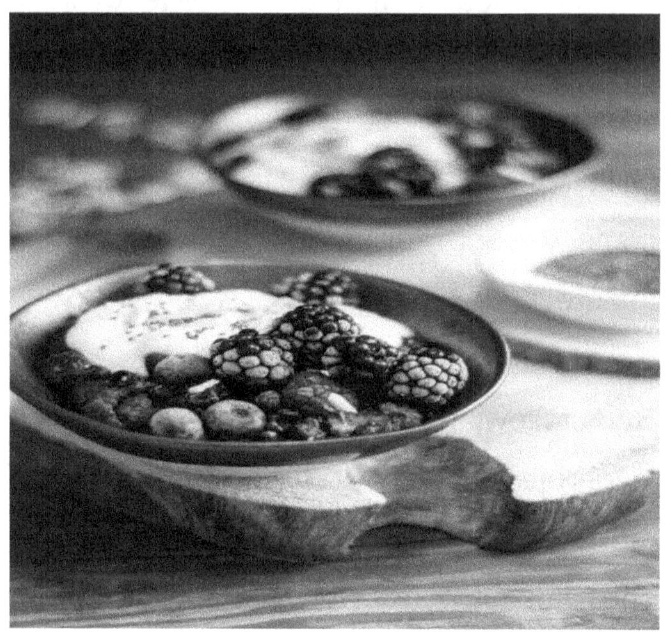

Berry almond crumble is a delightful and nutritious dessert option that aligns perfectly with the Blood Type O Diet. In this chapter, we explore how to create a delicious crumble using blood type O-friendly ingredients.

1. Choosing Blood Type O-Friendly Ingredients:

Select a variety of fresh or frozen berries such as strawberries, blueberries, raspberries, or blackberries as the main ingredient for your crumble. Berries are rich in antioxidants, vitamins, and fiber, making them an excellent choice for blood type O individuals. Opt for organic berries whenever possible for the best quality and nutritional value.

2. Incorporating Blood Type O-Friendly Sweeteners:

Sweeten your crumble with blood type O-friendly sweeteners such as honey, maple syrup, or coconut sugar. These natural sweeteners add sweetness to the crumble without the need for refined sugars or artificial sweeteners.

3. Adding Crunchy Almond Topping:

Create a crunchy topping for your crumble using blood type O-friendly ingredients such as almond flour, chopped almonds, rolled oats, and a touch of cinnamon. These ingredients add texture and flavor to the crumble while providing healthy fats and nutrients.

4. Balancing Flavors:

Balance the flavors of your berry almond crumble by adding a splash of lemon juice or zest to the berry filling. The acidity of the lemon helps to enhance the sweetness of the berries and create a more complex flavor profile.

5. Preparation Method:

Prepare the berry filling by tossing the berries with your chosen sweetener, lemon juice or zest, and a sprinkle of almond flour to thicken. Spread the berry mixture evenly in a baking dish and top with the almond crumble mixture.

6. Baking Instructions:

Bake the berry almond crumble in the oven at a moderate temperature (around 350°F or 175°C) until the berries are bubbly and the topping is golden brown and crispy. Allow the crumble to cool slightly before serving to allow the flavors to meld together.

7. Serving Suggestions:

Serve your berry almond crumble warm or at room temperature, garnished with a dollop of whipped coconut cream or a scoop of blood type O-friendly ice cream. This dessert can be enjoyed on its own or paired with a cup of herbal tea for a cozy treat.

8. Portion Control:

While berry almond crumble is a delicious dessert, it's important to practice portion control, especially if you're watching your calorie intake or trying to manage your weight. Enjoy a small serving of crumble as an occasional indulgence rather than a regular part of your diet.

9. Meal Prep and Storage Tips:
Prepare your berry almond crumble ahead of time and store leftovers in an airtight container in the refrigerator for up to several days. Reheat individual portions gently in the oven or microwave before serving to preserve their texture and flavor.

By following these guidelines and incorporating berry almond crumble into your diet, you can enjoy a flavorful and nutritious dessert that satisfies your sweet tooth while still supporting your health and well-being on the Blood Type O Diet.

Banana Walnut Cookies

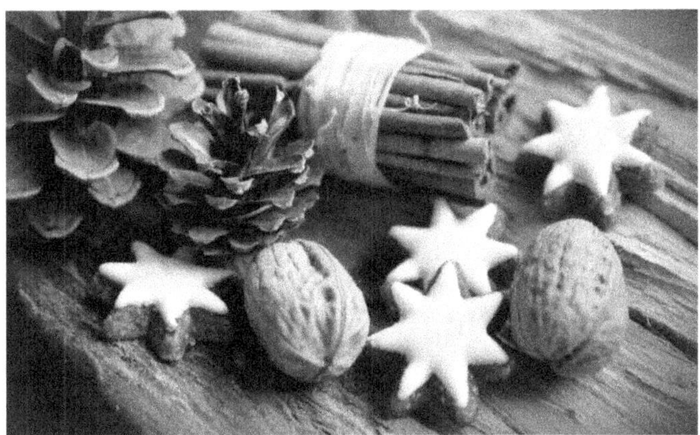

Banana walnut cookies offer a delicious and nutritious treat that is suitable for individuals following the Blood Type O Diet. In this chapter, we explore how to create these flavorful cookies using blood type O-friendly ingredients.

1. Choosing Blood Type O-Friendly Ingredients:

Select ripe bananas and walnuts as the main ingredients for your cookies. Bananas provide natural sweetness and moisture to the cookies, while walnuts add a crunchy texture and heart-healthy fats. Opt for organic bananas and walnuts whenever possible for the best quality and nutritional value.

2. Incorporating Blood Type O-Friendly Sweeteners:

Sweeten your cookies with blood type O-friendly sweeteners such as honey, maple syrup, or coconut sugar. These natural sweeteners add sweetness to the cookies without the need for refined sugars or artificial sweeteners.

3. Using Blood Type O-Friendly Flour Alternatives:

Replace traditional wheat flour with blood type O-friendly alternatives such as almond flour or coconut flour. These gluten-free flours provide a nutty flavor and a tender texture to the cookies while ensuring they are suitable for individuals with gluten sensitivities.

4. Adding Flavor and Texture:

Enhance the flavor of your banana walnut cookies by incorporating ingredients such as cinnamon, vanilla extract, and a pinch of salt. These additions add depth of flavor and help to balance the sweetness of the bananas and sweeteners.

5. Preparation Method:

Mash ripe bananas in a mixing bowl and stir in your chosen sweetener, flavorings, and any additional ingredients such as chopped walnuts or dark chocolate chips. Gradually add the flour until a thick batter forms, then scoop spoonfuls onto a baking sheet lined with parchment paper.

6. Baking Instructions:

Bake the banana walnut cookies in the oven at a moderate temperature (around 350°F or 175°C) until they are golden brown and firm to the touch, typically for about 10-12 minutes. Allow the cookies to cool on the baking sheet for a few minutes before transferring them to a wire rack to cool completely.

7. Serving Suggestions:

Serve your banana walnut cookies as a nutritious snack or dessert option, accompanied by a glass of unsweetened almond milk or herbal tea. These cookies can also be enjoyed as a quick breakfast on-the-go or as a post-workout energy boost.

8. Portion Control:

While banana walnut cookies are a healthier alternative to traditional cookies, it's important to practice portion control, especially if you're watching your calorie intake or trying to manage your weight. Enjoy a couple of cookies as a serving rather than indulging in the whole batch at once.

9. Meal Prep and Storage Tips:

Store your banana walnut cookies in an airtight container at room temperature for up to several days. For longer storage, freeze the cookies in a single layer on a baking sheet, then transfer them to a freezer-safe bag or container for up to a few months.

By following these guidelines and incorporating banana walnut cookies into your diet, you can enjoy a delicious and wholesome treat that satisfies your sweet cravings while still supporting your health and well-being on the Blood Type O Diet.

Chapter Nine: Beverages and Smoothies

Green Goddess Smoothie

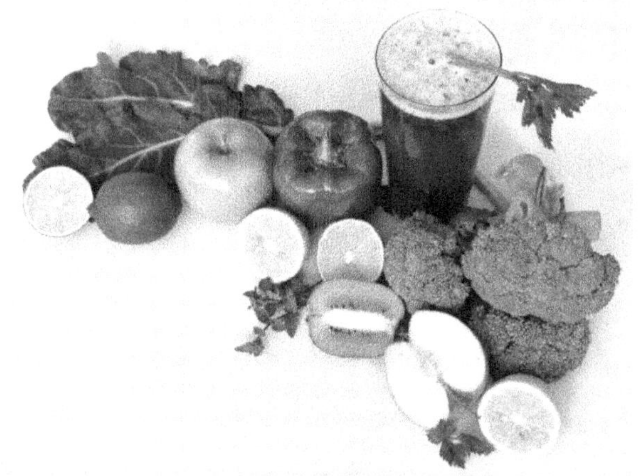

The Green Goddess Smoothie is a nutritious and refreshing beverage that perfectly aligns with the Blood Type O Diet. In this chapter, we explore how to create a delicious and nourishing smoothie using blood type O-friendly ingredients.

1. Choosing Blood Type O-Friendly Ingredients:

Select a variety of fresh, leafy greens such as spinach, kale, or Swiss chard as the base for your smoothie. These greens are rich in vitamins, minerals, and antioxidants, making them an excellent choice for blood type O individuals. Opt for organic greens whenever possible for the best quality and nutritional value.

2. Incorporating Blood Type O-Friendly Fruits:

Add blood type O-friendly fruits such as bananas, apples, or berries to your smoothie for natural sweetness and flavor. These fruits provide essential nutrients and fiber while complementing the earthy taste of the greens.

3. Adding Blood Type O-Friendly Protein:

Incorporate blood type O-friendly protein sources such as plain Greek yogurt, almond milk, or a scoop of protein powder into your smoothie. Protein helps to keep you feeling full and satisfied while supporting muscle repair and growth.

4. Using Healthy Fats:

Include blood type O-friendly fats such as avocado, chia seeds, or flaxseed oil in your smoothie to provide satiety and promote heart health. These fats add creaminess to the smoothie and help to balance blood sugar levels.

5. Balancing Flavors and Textures:

Balance the flavors and textures of your Green Goddess Smoothie by experimenting with different combinations of ingredients. Consider adding a splash of citrus juice, a sprinkle of cinnamon, or a handful of nuts or seeds for added crunch and flavor.

6. Preparation Method:

Combine your chosen leafy greens, fruits, protein source, healthy fats, and any additional ingredients in a blender. Blend on high speed until smooth and creamy, adding water or ice as needed to achieve your desired consistency.

7. Customizing to Suit Individual Preferences:

The Green Goddess Smoothie is highly customizable, allowing individuals to tailor ingredients and flavors to their liking. Feel free to adjust the ratios of greens to fruits, or experiment with different combinations of ingredients to create your perfect smoothie.

8. Serving Suggestions:

Enjoy your Green Goddess Smoothie as a nutrient-rich breakfast option, a post-workout recovery drink, or a refreshing afternoon snack. Serve the smoothie in a glass or portable bottle for on-the-go convenience.

9. Portion Control:

While Green Goddess Smoothies are a healthy choice, it's important to practice portion control, especially if you're watching your calorie intake or trying to manage your weight. Enjoy a single serving of smoothie as part of a balanced meal or snack.

10. Meal Prep and Storage Tips:

Prepare a batch of Green Goddess Smoothie ahead of time and store individual servings in airtight containers or freezer-safe bags in the refrigerator or freezer for quick and convenient meals throughout the week.

Thaw frozen smoothie portions in the refrigerator overnight or blend with a splash of water or milk to refresh.

By following these guidelines and incorporating Green Goddess Smoothies into your diet, you can enjoy a delicious and nutrient-packed beverage that supports your health and well-being on the Blood Type O Diet.

Hibiscus Iced Tea

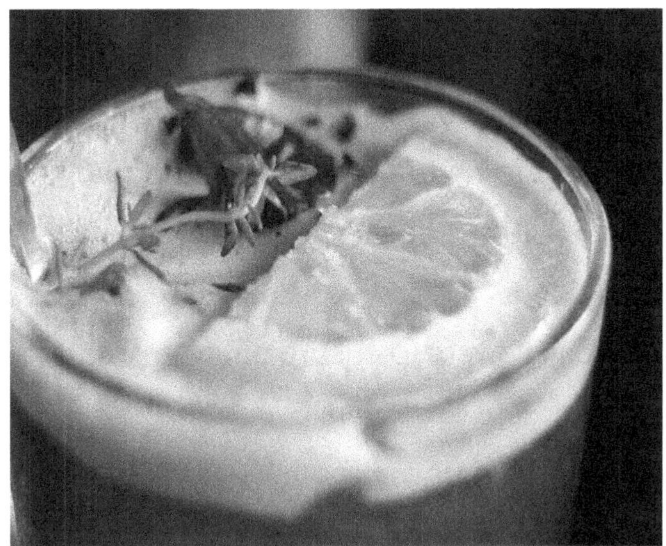

Hibiscus iced tea is a refreshing and flavorful beverage that is not only delicious but also aligns well with the Blood Type O Diet. In this chapter, we explore how to create a vibrant and hydrating hibiscus tea using blood type O-friendly ingredients.

1. Choosing Blood Type O-Friendly Ingredients:

Start with high-quality dried hibiscus flowers as the main ingredient for your tea. Hibiscus flowers are rich in antioxidants and have a tangy, floral flavor that makes for a refreshing beverage. Look for organic hibiscus flowers to ensure purity and quality.

2. Incorporating Blood Type O-Friendly Sweeteners:

Sweeten your hibiscus iced tea with blood type O-friendly sweeteners such as honey, maple syrup, or stevia. These natural sweeteners add sweetness to the tea without the need for refined sugars or artificial sweeteners.

3. Adding Flavor Enhancements:

Enhance the flavor of your hibiscus tea by incorporating ingredients such as fresh ginger, lemon or orange slices, or a few sprigs of mint. These additions add complexity to the flavor profile of the tea and create a refreshing and aromatic beverage.

4. Brewing Method:

To brew hibiscus iced tea, bring water to a boil in a saucepan and then remove it from the heat. Add dried hibiscus flowers to the hot water and steep for about 10-15 minutes, depending on desired strength. Strain the tea into a pitcher and allow it to cool to room temperature before refrigerating.

5. Serving Suggestions:

Serve your hibiscus iced tea chilled over ice, garnished with fresh fruit slices, mint leaves, or edible flowers for an elegant touch. This tea is perfect for enjoying on a hot day or as a refreshing beverage with meals.

6. Customizing to Suit Individual Preferences:

Hibiscus iced tea is highly customizable, allowing individuals to tailor the flavor and sweetness to their liking. Experiment with different combinations of sweeteners and flavorings to create your perfect cup of tea.

7. Benefits for Blood Type O Individuals:

Hibiscus tea offers several health benefits that are particularly advantageous for blood type O individuals. It supports cardiovascular health, aids digestion, and helps to regulate blood sugar levels, making it a valuable addition to the diet.

8. Hydration and Antioxidants:

In addition to its refreshing taste, hibiscus iced tea provides hydration and a dose of antioxidants, which help to combat oxidative stress and inflammation in the body. Staying hydrated and consuming antioxidant-rich beverages like hibiscus tea can support overall health and well-being.

9. Portion Control:

While hibiscus iced tea is a healthy beverage choice, it's important to practice portion control, especially if you're watching your calorie intake or trying to manage your weight. Enjoy a single serving of tea as part of a balanced diet.

10. Meal Pairing Suggestions:

Pair your hibiscus iced tea with light and refreshing dishes such as salads, grilled fish, or fruit salads. The tangy and floral notes of the tea complement a wide variety of flavors and cuisines.

By following these guidelines and incorporating hibiscus iced tea into your diet, you can enjoy a delicious and hydrating beverage that supports your health and well-being on the Blood Type O Diet.

Berry Blast Protein Shake

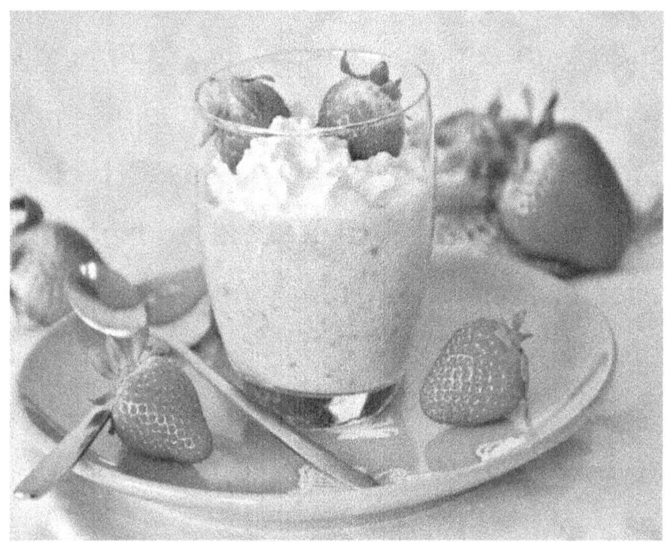

The Berry Blast Protein Shake is a delicious and nutrient-packed beverage that is ideal for individuals following the Blood Type O Diet. In this chapter, we explore how to create a satisfying and energizing protein shake using blood type O-friendly ingredients.

1. Choosing Blood Type O-Friendly Ingredients:

Start with a base of blood type O-friendly protein powder, such as pea protein or rice protein isolate. These plant-based protein sources are easily digestible and provide essential amino acids for muscle repair and growth.

2. Incorporating Blood Type O-Friendly Fruits:

Add a variety of blood type O-friendly berries to your protein shake for natural sweetness and antioxidant benefits. Berries such as strawberries, blueberries, raspberries, and blackberries are rich in vitamins, minerals, and fiber, making them an excellent addition to the shake.

3. Using Blood Type O-Friendly Liquid Base:

Choose a blood type O-friendly liquid base for your protein shake, such as unsweetened almond milk, coconut milk, or water. These options are low in calories and carbohydrates, making them suitable for individuals following the Blood Type O Diet.

4. Adding Healthy Fats:

Incorporate blood type O-friendly fats into your protein shake for added satiety and nutrient absorption. Options include avocado, almond butter, or a tablespoon of flaxseed oil. These fats help to balance blood sugar levels and keep you feeling full for longer.

5. Balancing Flavors and Textures:

Balance the flavors and textures of your Berry Blast Protein Shake by experimenting with different combinations of ingredients. Consider adding a handful of spinach or kale for added nutrients and a creamy texture, or a dash of cinnamon or vanilla extract for extra flavor.

6. Preparation Method:
Combine your chosen protein powder, berries, liquid base, healthy fats, and any additional ingredients in a blender. Blend on high speed until smooth and creamy, adding more liquid if needed to achieve your desired consistency.

7. Customizing to Suit Individual Preferences:

The Berry Blast Protein Shake is highly customizable, allowing individuals to tailor the flavor and sweetness to their liking. Adjust the ratios of ingredients to suit your taste preferences, or experiment with different types of protein powders and fruits for variety.

8. Serving Suggestions:

Enjoy your Berry Blast Protein Shake as a post-workout recovery drink, a quick and nutritious breakfast option, or a satisfying afternoon snack. Serve the shake in a glass or portable bottle for on-the-go convenience.

9. Portion Control:

While protein shakes can be a convenient and nutritious option, it's important to practice portion control, especially if you're watching your calorie intake or trying to manage your weight. Enjoy a single serving of the shake as part of a balanced meal or snack.

10. Meal Pairing Suggestions:

Pair your Berry Blast Protein Shake with a small serving of protein-rich foods such as grilled chicken, tofu, or hard-boiled eggs for a complete and balanced meal. Alternatively, enjoy the shake alongside a handful of nuts or seeds for added texture and flavor.

By following these guidelines and incorporating Berry Blast Protein Shakes into your diet, you can enjoy a delicious and satisfying beverage that supports your health and well-being on the Blood Type O Diet.

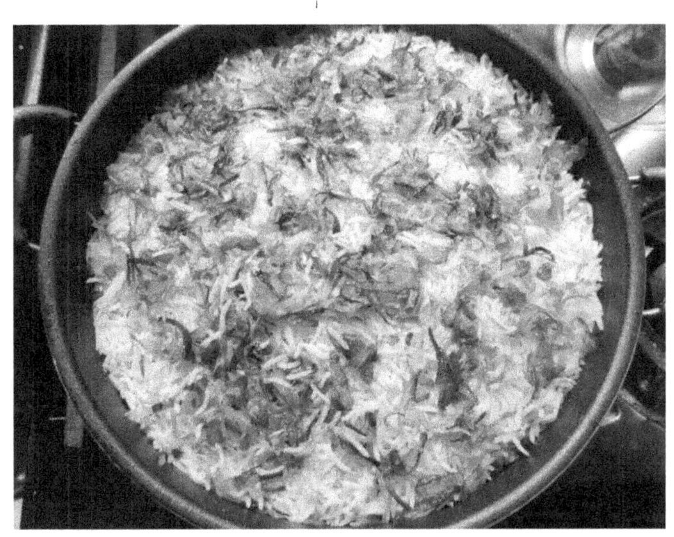

Chapter Ten: Special Occasion Meals

Grilled Steak with Chimichurri Sauce

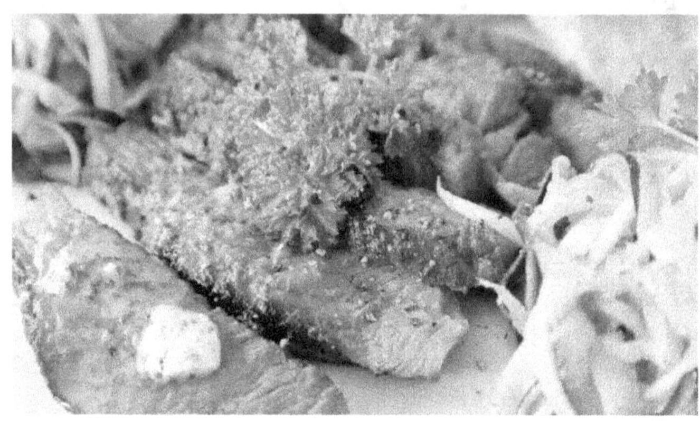

Grilled steak with chimichurri sauce is a flavorful and satisfying dish that perfectly fits the Blood Type O Diet. In this chapter, we explore how to create a delicious and nutrient-rich meal using blood type O-friendly ingredients.

1. Choosing Blood Type O-Friendly Steak:

Select a lean cut of beef such as sirloin, flank, or skirt steak for your grilled steak. These cuts are rich in protein and iron, making them an excellent choice for blood type O individuals. Opt for grass-fed or organic beef whenever possible for the best quality and nutritional value.

2. Incorporating Blood Type O-Friendly Herbs and Spices:

Prepare a chimichurri sauce using blood type O-friendly herbs and spices such as parsley, cilantro, garlic, oregano, and red pepper flakes. These herbs and spices add flavor and depth to the dish without the need for added salt or artificial seasonings.

3. Using Healthy Cooking Methods:

Grill your steak using a healthy cooking method such as grilling or broiling. Avoid frying or deep-frying, as these methods can add unnecessary calories and unhealthy fats to the dish. Grilling allows excess fat to drip away from the meat, resulting in a leaner and healthier meal.

4. Balancing Flavors and Textures:

Balance the flavors and textures of your grilled steak by marinating it in a mixture of olive oil, garlic, and lemon juice before grilling. This marinade adds moisture and flavor to the steak while tenderizing the meat for a juicy and delicious result.

5. Preparing Chimichurri Sauce:

Prepare chimichurri sauce by combining chopped herbs, minced garlic, olive oil, red wine vinegar, and a pinch of salt and pepper in a bowl. Allow the flavors to meld together for at least 30 minutes before serving to enhance the taste of the sauce.

6. Serving Suggestions:

Serve your grilled steak with chimichurri sauce alongside a side of roasted vegetables, a fresh salad, or a serving of whole grains such as quinoa or brown rice. The bright and tangy flavors of the chimichurri sauce complement the richness of the steak and add freshness to the dish.

7. Portion Control:

While steak is a nutritious protein source, it's important to practice portion control, especially if you're watching your calorie intake or trying to manage your weight. Aim for a serving of steak that is about the size of your palm, and fill the rest of your plate with vegetables and whole grains.

8. Meal Pairing Suggestions:

Pair your grilled steak with chimichurri sauce with a glass of red wine or sparkling water infused with citrus slices for a refreshing and enjoyable meal. Consider adding a side of grilled asparagus, sautéed mushrooms, or roasted sweet potatoes for added variety and nutrition.

By following these guidelines and incorporating grilled steak with chimichurri sauce into your diet, you can enjoy a delicious and satisfying meal that supports your health and well-being on the Blood Type O Diet.

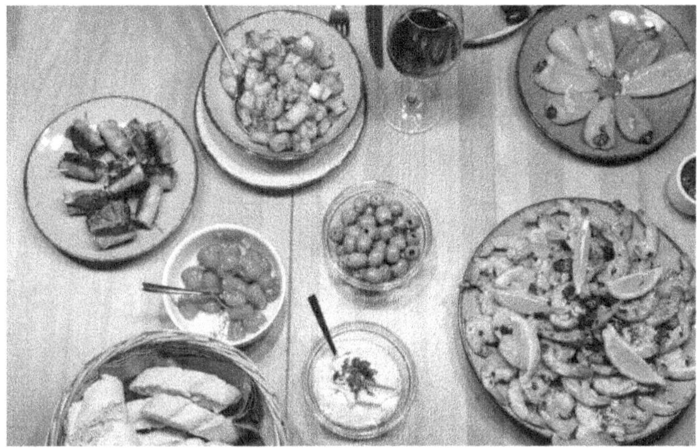

Shrimp and veggie skewers offer a delicious and nutritious option for individuals following the Blood Type O Diet. In this chapter, we explore how to create flavorful and balanced skewers using blood type O-friendly ingredients.

1. Choosing Blood Type O-Friendly Ingredients:

Select fresh shrimp as the main protein source for your skewers. Shrimp is low in fat and calories, high in protein, and rich in essential nutrients such as iodine and selenium, making it an excellent choice for blood type O individuals. Opt for wild-caught shrimp whenever possible for the best quality and flavor.

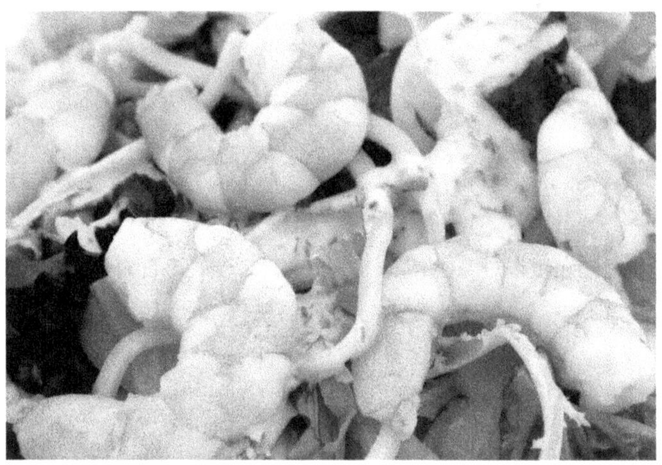

2. Incorporating Blood Type O-Friendly Vegetables:

Add a variety of blood type O-friendly vegetables to your skewers for color, flavor, and added nutrition. Some options include bell peppers, zucchini, cherry tomatoes, mushrooms, and onions. These vegetables provide vitamins, minerals, and fiber, enhancing the nutritional value of the skewers.

3. Using Healthy Cooking Methods:

Grill or broil your shrimp and veggie skewers using a healthy cooking method that minimizes added fats and calories. Grilling allows the flavors of the ingredients to meld together while imparting a delicious smoky char. Avoid frying or deep-frying, as these methods can add unnecessary calories and unhealthy fats to the dish.

4. Balancing Flavors:

Balance the flavors of your shrimp and veggie skewers by marinating the shrimp in a mixture of olive oil, lemon juice, garlic, and herbs such as parsley, thyme, and oregano. This marinade adds moisture and flavor to the shrimp while complementing the natural sweetness of the vegetables.

5. Assembling the Skewers:

Thread the marinated shrimp and vegetables onto skewers, alternating between the shrimp and vegetables to ensure even cooking. Leave a small space between each ingredient to allow for even heat distribution and thorough cooking.

6. Grilling Instructions:

Preheat your grill to medium-high heat and lightly oil the grates to prevent sticking. Place the skewers on the grill and cook for 2-3 minutes per side, or until the shrimp are opaque and the vegetables are tender-crisp. Be careful not to overcook the shrimp, as they can become rubbery and tough.

7. Serving Suggestions:

Serve your shrimp and veggie skewers hot off the grill, garnished with a sprinkle of fresh herbs such as chopped parsley or basil. These skewers can be enjoyed as a main course alongside a side of whole grains or a fresh salad, or as a flavorful appetizer for gatherings and parties.

8. Portion Control:

While shrimp and veggie skewers are a nutritious option, it's important to practice portion control, especially if you're watching your calorie intake or trying to manage your weight. Aim for a serving size that includes a moderate portion of shrimp and vegetables, and fill the rest of your plate with additional vegetables or whole grains.

9. Meal Pairing Suggestions:

Pair your shrimp and veggie skewers with a light and refreshing side dish such as quinoa salad, grilled asparagus, or cucumber salad with a lemon vinaigrette. These dishes complement the flavors of the skewers and add variety to the meal.

By following these guidelines and incorporating shrimp and veggie skewers into your diet, you can enjoy a delicious and nutritious meal that supports your health and well-being on the Blood Type O Diet.

Vegetarian Zucchini Lasagna

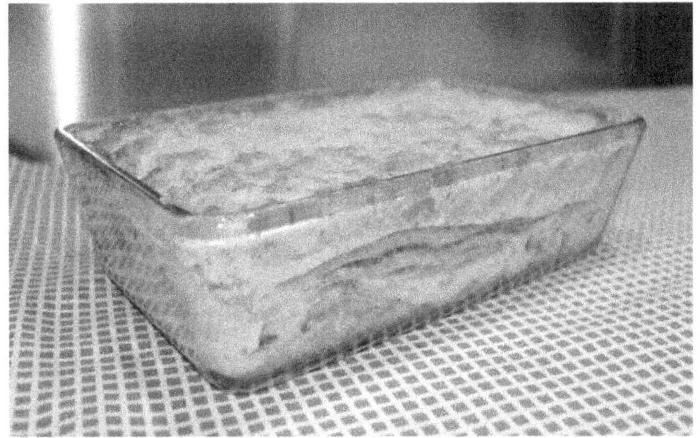

Vegetarian zucchini lasagna offers a delicious and nutritious twist on the classic Italian dish that perfectly fits the Blood Type O Diet. In this chapter, we explore how to create a flavorful and satisfying lasagna using blood type O-friendly ingredients.

1. Choosing Blood Type O-Friendly Ingredients:

Select fresh zucchini as the main ingredient for your lasagna noodles. Zucchini is low in calories and carbohydrates, rich in vitamins and minerals, and provides a light and refreshing alternative to traditional pasta noodles. Opt for organic zucchini whenever possible for the best quality and flavor.

2. Incorporating Blood Type O-Friendly Protein Sources:

Add blood type O-friendly protein sources such as tofu, lentils, or black beans to your lasagna filling. These plant-based proteins provide essential amino acids and nutrients while keeping the dish light and satisfying. Experiment with different protein sources to find your favorite combination.

3. Using Blood Type O-Friendly Cheeses:

Choose blood type O-friendly cheeses such as goat cheese, feta cheese, or mozzarella cheese for your lasagna. These cheeses are lower in lactose and easier to digest than other dairy products, making them suitable for individuals with lactose intolerance. Use cheese in moderation to avoid excessive saturated fat intake.

4. Incorporating Blood Type O-Friendly Vegetables:

Layer your lasagna with a variety of blood type O-friendly vegetables such as bell peppers, onions, spinach, mushrooms, and tomatoes. These vegetables add flavor, texture, and essential nutrients to the dish while keeping it light and nutritious.

5. Balancing Flavors and Textures:

Balance the flavors and textures of your vegetarian zucchini lasagna by layering the ingredients with a rich and flavorful tomato sauce. Season the sauce with herbs and spices such as basil, oregano, garlic, and red pepper flakes to enhance the taste of the lasagna without the need for added salt or artificial seasonings.

6. Assembling the Lasagna:

Layer the zucchini noodles, protein source, vegetables, cheese, and tomato sauce in a baking dish, repeating the layers until all ingredients are used. Top the lasagna with a final layer of cheese and a sprinkle of herbs for added flavor and visual appeal.

7. Baking Instructions:

Bake the vegetarian zucchini lasagna in the oven at a moderate temperature (around 375°F or 190°C) until the cheese is melted and bubbly and the edges are golden brown, typically for about 30-40 minutes. Allow the lasagna to cool slightly before slicing and serving.

8. Serving Suggestions:

Serve your vegetarian zucchini lasagna hot out of the oven, garnished with fresh basil or parsley for a pop of color and freshness. This lasagna pairs well with a side salad dressed with a light vinaigrette or a serving of steamed vegetables for added nutrition.

9. Portion Control:

While vegetarian zucchini lasagna is a lighter and healthier alternative to traditional lasagna, it's important to practice portion control, especially if you're watching your calorie intake or trying to manage your weight. Enjoy a single serving of lasagna as part of a balanced meal.

10. Meal Pairing Suggestions:

Pair your vegetarian zucchini lasagna with a glass of red wine or sparkling water infused with citrus slices for a refreshing and enjoyable meal. Consider adding a side of garlic bread or roasted potatoes for added comfort and satisfaction.

By following these guidelines and incorporating vegetarian zucchini lasagna into your diet, you can enjoy a delicious and nutritious meal that supports your health and well-being on the Blood Type O Diet.

Conclusion

As we conclude our journey through "The Blood Type O Diet Cookbook," we've explored a diverse array of flavorful and nutritious recipes tailored specifically for individuals with blood type O. Throughout this cookbook, we've delved into the principles of the Blood Type O Diet, emphasizing the importance of consuming foods that align with your blood type to optimize health and well-being.

By focusing on blood type O-friendly ingredients and culinary techniques, we've discovered how to create delicious meals that not only satisfy the palate but also support overall health and vitality. From energizing smoothie bowls to hearty breakfast hashes, grilled protein dishes to vibrant salads, and decadent desserts to refreshing beverages, each recipe has been carefully crafted to provide nourishment and enjoyment while adhering to the principles of the Blood Type O Diet.

Throughout our culinary exploration, we've emphasized the importance of incorporating a variety of nutrient-dense foods into your diet, including lean proteins, fruits, vegetables, healthy fats, and whole grains. By embracing a diverse and balanced approach to eating, individuals with blood type O can support optimal digestion, metabolism, and immune function while reducing the risk of chronic disease and promoting overall well-being.

As you continue your diet with the Blood Type O Diet, remember to listen to your body's unique needs and preferences. Pay attention to how different foods make you feel and adjust your dietary choices accordingly. Experiment with new ingredients, flavors, and cooking methods to keep your meals exciting and enjoyable.

Above all, approach your dietary journey with curiosity, mindfulness, and a sense of adventure. By nourishing your body with wholesome, blood type O-friendly foods, you're taking an important step towards achieving optimal health and vitality for years to come.

Thank you for joining us on this culinary exploration of the Blood Type O Diet. May these recipes inspire you to embrace the power of food as a tool for health, happiness, and vitality. Here's to your continued well-being and culinary adventures ahead.